DORA – HYSTERIA – GENDER
Reconsidering Freud's Case Study

FIGURES OF THE UNCONSCIOUS 16

Editorial Board
Jeffrey Bloechl (Boston College), Gilson Iannini (Universidade Federal de Ouro Preto), Beatriz Santos (Paris), Philippe Van Haute (Radboud Universiteit, Nijmegen)

Advisory Board
Lisa Baraitser (Birkbeck College, London), Rudolf Bernet (KU Leuven), Rachel Blass (Heythrop College, London), Guillaume Sibertin-Blanc (Université Toulouse II - Le Mirail), Richard Boothby (Loyola University, Maryland), Marcus Coelen (Ludwig-Maximilians-Universität, München), Jozef Corveleyn (KU Leuven), Monique David-Ménard (Université Paris VII - Diderot), Rodrigo De La Fabián (Universidad Diego Portales, Santiago de Chile), Jens De Vleminck (Leuven), Eran Dorfman (University of Tel Aviv), Tomas Geyskens (Leuven), Patrick Guyomard (Université Paris VII - Diderot), Ari Hirvonen (University of Helsinki), Laurie Laufer (Université Paris VII - Diderot), Paul Moyaert (KU Leuven), Elissa Marder (Emory University, Atlanta), Paola Marrati (Johns Hopkins University), Claire Nioche (Université Paris XIII), Claudio Oliveira (Universidade Federal Fluminense), Guilherme Massara Rocha (Universidade Federal de Minas Gerais), Elizabeth Rottenberg (De Paul University, Chicago), Vladimir Safatle (Universidade de São Paulo), Stella Sandford (Kingston College), Charles Shepherdson (State University of New York at Albany), Celine Surprenant (Paris), Antônio Teixeira (Universidade Federal de Minas Gerais), Patrick Vandermeersch (University of Groningen), Johan Van Der Walt (University of Luxemburg), Veronica Vasterling (Radboud Universiteit, Nijmegen), Wilfried Ver Eecke, (Georgetown University), Jamieson Webster (The New School, New York), Herman Westerink (Radboud Universiteit, Nijmegen)

DORA – HYSTERIA – GENDER

Reconsidering Freud's Case Study

A Sigmund Freud Museum's Symposium

Edited by
Daniela Finzi & Herman Westerink

LEUVEN UNIVERSITY PRESS

This publication has been financially supported by the
Vienna Municipal Department of Cultural Affairs (MA7)

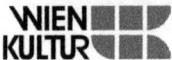

and the Sigmund Freud Foundation

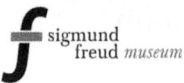

© 2018 by Leuven University Press / Universitaire Pers Leuven / Presses Universitaires de Louvain.
Minderbroedersstraat 4, B-3000 Leuven (Belgium)

All rights reserved. Except in those cases expressly determined by law, no part of this publication may be multiplied, saved in an automated datafile or made public in any way whatsoever without the express prior written consent of the publishers.

ISBN 978 94 6270 156 4
e-ISBN 978 94 6166 261 3
D/2018/1869/37
NUR: 777, 730

Cover design: Griet Van Haute
Lay-out: Friedemann bvba

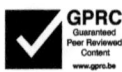

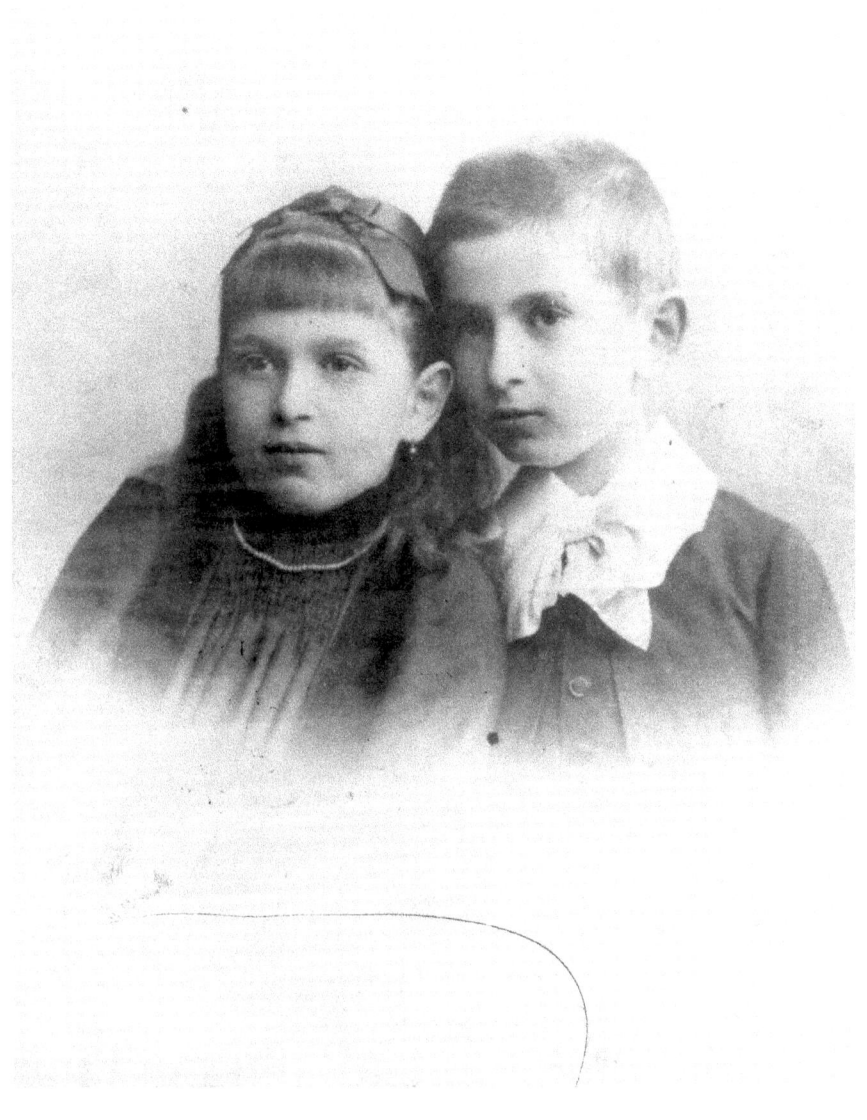

Ida and Otto Bauer as children, 1890
Courtesy: Verein für Geschichte der ArbeiterInnenbewegung, Vienna

Table of Contents

Preface
Monika Pessler … 9

Introduction
Daniela Finzi and Herman Westerink … 11

Narrative Strategies and Hermeneutic Desire:
Constructions of a Case History
Daniela Finzi … 17

The Analytic Denial of Freud's Struggle with the
Understanding of Dora: Simplifying the Oedipus Complex
and the Process of its Adoption
Rachel B. Blass … 33

Sexuality and Knowledge in Dora's Case
Beatriz Santos … 45

Trauma and Disgust:
Dora between Freud and Laplanche
Philippe Van Haute … 59

Sucking, Kissing and Disgust –
Dora and the Theory of Infantile Sexuality
Herman Westerink … 73

Dora, the Un-Ending and ever Unraveling Story
Jeanne Wolff Bernstein … 89

On the Signification of Dora's Father
Ulrike Kadi … 101

From Dora to Conchita:
Recent Views on Gender and Sexuality in Psychoanalysis
Ilka Quindeau   115

The Case of Dora –
A Queer Perspective on Hysteria and Perversion
Esther Hutfless   135

Notes on the Contributors   149

Preface

Since the Dora's case study was published at the beginning of the last century, it has not only been regarded as a watershed in the history of psychoanalysis. Freud's detailed description of his ultimately 'failed' treatment of the young hysteric patient Ida Bauer, who eluded the psychoanalyst by breaking off the therapy after just a few months, still offers a kaleidoscopic array of socially and politically relevant references. In addition to practical phenomena of psychoanalysis such as the potential of transference, Freud's account of female sexual development equally raises a number of questions pertaining to social and cultural theory. Commensurately, the authors of this publication approach the complexity of this text and the ambivalent history of its reception from different perspectives – psychoanalytic and specifically cultural views of literary research, gender and queer studies illuminate this fragmentary work that has from the outset prompted critical scrutiny. Drawing on the historical knowledge gain that acknowledged the potential for a meaningful new beginning even in failure, the publication presents a timely scientific discourse in an interplay of correlating disciplines – for which I would like to thank everyone involved, our cooperation partners and the authors.

Monika Pessler
Director
Sigmund Freud Museum, Vienna

Introduction

From Sigmund Freud's correspondence with Wilhelm Fliess we know that he started the treatment of the seventeen-year-old Ida Bauer – 'Dora' – in the second half of 1900. Ida Bauer was born in Vienna on November 1, 1882, into a bourgeois Bohemian-Jewish family. Together with her parents and her brother Otto, who would later become a social democratic politician and a key figure in the Austro-Marxist movement, the family moved to a village near Meran (South Tyrol) in 1888. They moved back to Vienna in 1900, only a few months before Ida started her treatment with Freud. The family lived in Freud's neighborhood. The treatment of 'Dora' lasted only three months, as it was broken off at the patient's wish on December 31, 1900.

Immediately afterwards, Freud started writing the case study which he intended to give the title 'Dream and Hysteria'. This original title indicates the objectives Freud had in view. On the one hand, Freud wished this case study to be a supplement to *The Interpretation of Dreams* published only a year before in November 1899. For this reason, Freud had grouped the material around two dreams that are indeed at the heart of the case study as we know it. On the other hand, Freud wished to stimulate interest in the complexity of psychological events in the clinical phenomenon of hysteria – a complexity that was brought to light in the psychoanalytic clinical practice. 'Dream and Hysteria' was composed with the aim of substantiating the views upon the pathogenesis of hysterical symptoms and certain psychic processes Freud had already put forward in his earlier texts on hysteria from 1895 and 1896, he writes in the first paragraph of the 'Prefatory Remarks' to the case study.

The original aim of the case study thus seems to have been to further investigate two grand topics Freud had been working on in the 1890s: the analysis and treatment of hysteria and the interpretation of dreams. The case study was intended to bring these two lines of research together by showing the clinical relevance of dream interpretation for the discovery of the repressed aspects of psychic life. Dream interpretation would help to further refine the psychoanalytic techniques. But there was more. On a fundamental level, Freud's interest in dream analysis was triggered by a clinical problem: the unresolved question of the mechanisms involved in hysterical symptom formation. Freud had high hopes that the analyses of a generally human phenomenon such as dreams would give valuable insight in the etiology of hysteria--that is, in the juxtaposition of ideas and tendencies, the repression of ideas, the displacement of affects (excitation) and the conversion of these affects into physically manifested symptoms. In the 'Prefatory Remarks' to the case study, Freud remarks on the case not providing answers for all of the questions arising out of the problems of hysteria: "It is not fair to expect from a single case more than it can offer".[1] In this sense the case study was 'incomplete'. Freud did not deliver a systematic discussion of all possible kinds of relations between dreams and hysteria. According to Freud himself, this was one the reasons why the case study remained a 'fragment' and was only eventually published in November 1905 under the title 'Fragment of an Analysis of a Case of Hysteria'. Another major reason for the case study being 'incomplete' and fragmented was the fact that the analysis was broken off by Dora and not carried through to its proper end.

We know that Freud sent the manuscript of 'Dream and Hysteria' to the *Monatschrift für Psychiatrie und Neurologie* in 1901. It was accepted for publication, but for unknown reasons Freud reconsidered the publication of the text. In 1904, he submitted the manuscript to the editor of the *Journal für Psychologie und Neurologie* – a journal based at the famous Burghölzli clinic where Freud expected to meet a friendly audience (notably in the figure of Eugen Bleuler). The editor, Korbinian Brodmann, however, rejected the manuscript. Freud then decided to publish the 'Fragment' in two parts in the 1905 October and November issues of *Monatschrift für Psychiatrie und Neurologie* since it had been accepted already three years before.[2]

This publication in 1905 was no coincidence. Freud had good reasons to make the text available shortly after another major text had been published, *Three Essays on the Theory of Sexuality*. One could argue that implicitly the 'Fragment' was no longer only intended to be a case study on dream and hysteria, but in fact became a supplement to *Three Essays* substantiating some of the major claims in that text. Whatever the exact mechanism in the formation of symptoms, one thing that is clear is that "the symptoms of the disease are nothing else than *the patient's sexual activity*", Freud writes in the 'Postscript' to 'Fragment'.[3] That is to say, these symptoms not only draw strength from repressed 'normal' sexuality but much more from unconscious perverse activities. The hysteric's unconscious phantasies show exactly the same content as the actions of perverts,

---

[1] S. Freud, 'Fragment of an Analysis of a Case of Hysteria', Standard Edition 7, J. Strachey (Ed.). London: Hogarth Press, 1953, p. 13. In this volume all authors will reference the Standard Edition (SE), unless explicitly mentioned otherwise.
[2] On the publication history of the Dora case see, T.A. Tanner, 'Sigmund Freud und die Zeitschrift für Hypnotismus', *Luzifer-Amor* 18 (2005-36), pp. 65-118.
[3] S. Freud, 'Fragment', p. 115.

Freud remarks in the Dora case, and it is this relation between hysteria and perversion that is also at the very center of *Three Essays*.

The 'Fragment' is thus certainly not merely a last – maybe too late – case of hysteria that connects to the actual *Studies on Hysteria* from 1895, linking Dora to the other female hysteric patients – Katharina, Emma, Elisabeth, and others. It is a key publication written in a period in which Freud lays the foundation for psychoanalysis as both practice and theory. It is a case study in which Freud explores three interrelated topics: hysteria, sexuality, and dreams. Together with *Three Essays* the Dora case is also the last grand study on hysteria – and as such it marks the end of an era. After 1905 Freud will turn his attention to other psychopathologies – obsessional neurosis, paranoia and melancholia – that will determine the further course of the development of psychoanalytic theory.

Given the fragmented nature of the text, its ties to other fundamental psychoanalytic texts and topics, and its place in the development of Freudian psychoanalysis and in his oeuvre, it can hardly be called surprising that the Dora case has produced very different readings from different perspectives focusing on different aspects of the text – hysteria, dreams, trauma, transference, homosexuality/bisexuality, adolescence, gender, the text's genre, et cetera. This volume connects to this history of readings and a body of literature on the Dora case. This volume displays very different readings of the 'Fragment' from a variety of perspectives. The lack of consensus should, however, not be seen as a shortcoming or failure, but, quite to the contrary, as a productive state of affairs making visible fundamental problems in Freud's writings and the interpretation of his writings. In that sense, this volume mirrors the incompleteness of 'Fragment' itself.

What then are the fundamental problems in Freudian thought addressed in the text and/or the literature on the text? As we have already said, the case study was intended to shed light on the pathogenesis of hysterical symptom formation, and as such on the etiology of hysteria as such. As regards the latter issue, the text raises important questions about the role of constitutional (hereditary) and accidental (traumatic) factors in this etiology. This is a fundamental problem addressed by Freud in many of his clinical and theoretical writings. It is – more importantly – also a problem that is closely related to various interpretations of the development of Freudian theory. Did Freud abandon the so-called seduction theory (accidental factors) in favor of a theory highlighting constitution? Or was there in fact much more continuity – as Freud seems to suggest in the opening sentences of the 'Prefatory Remarks'? Another fundamental problem concerns the connection to the 1905 *Three Essays* – a text in which Freud presented a non-Oedipal theory of infantile sexuality very much inspired by his insights in Dora's hysteria. If Freud underscores the infantile sexuality as being autoerotic and without object, how then should the 'Fragment' be read? Is it an Oedipal tale, a 'family romance' spinning around object relations and Oedipal phantasies? Or is it, to the contrary, an elaboration of the constitutional aspects that structure Dora's infantile life, and which only later – in puberty – becomes associated with objects? Is the Dora case the first clinical evidence of an Oedipus complex, or is it actually a perfect substantiation and illustration of a non-Oedipal theory of infantile sexuality? Another set of questions concerns issues related to femininity – the transference in Freud's treatment of a feminine patient, the character of feminine sexuality, the position of female persons in a bourgeois Viennese family, bisexual and lesbian desire, et cetera.

This volume does not aim at solving problems or finding consensus. With this volume, we intend to articulate and explore these problems and questions in their complexity in order to open a space again for new readings of Freud's texts and new views on the development of Freudian theory.

This volume brings together papers that – for the majority – were presented at a conference entitled 'Dora – Hysteria – Gender' organized by the Sigmund Freud Foundation (Vienna) in cooperation with the Freud Research Group (International Society for Psychoanalysis and Philosophy) at the Berggasse 19 in 2016 – the house where Dora was analyzed and where she lived just around the corner at the Liechtensteinstrasse.

In the first contribution, 'Narrative Strategies and Hermeneutic Desire. Constructions of a Case History', Daniela Finzi reads Freud's case history as a narrative text, tackling it with the instruments of literary analysis and asking for its hermeneutic dynamics. The theoretical discussion about the Dora case's place in psychoanalytic theory is introduced by the next contributor, Rachel Blass. Starting from the common critiques regarding Freud's alleged Oedipal interpretations, Blass demonstrates in 'The Analytical Denial of Freud's Struggle with the Understanding of Dora' to which extent these claims are plausible, given the fact that, in her opinion, Freud doesn't offer any Oedipal interpretation in the Dora case. Blass doesn't merely criticize these readings, but also explores the motives behind these readings. Beatriz Santos in her contribution raises the question of Freud's knowledge of sexuality and, more specific, of the hysterical disposition in the Dora case and the writings preceding that case study. She argues that the case study is both clinically and theoretically a 'work on fragments'. In a familiar way, Philippe Van Haute tackles the tradition of interpreting the Dora case along Oedipal lines, arguing for a non-Oedipal reading of the text while exploring the theory of trauma as presented in the case. Herman Westerink, in his chapter 'Sucking, Kissing and Disgust – Dora and the Theory of Infantile Sexuality', situates the Dora case in the context of the texts which are strongly related to the 'Fragment': *The Interpretation of Dreams* and the *Three Essays*, but also Freud's writings on hysteria from the 1890s. Focussing on the issue of oral sexuality in the Dora case, he comes to the conclusion that Freud's young patient served as a model for the theory of infantile sexuality presented in *Three Essays*. Jeanne Wolff Bernstein, from a Lacanian perspective, in her article 'Dora, the Un-Ending and ever Unraveling Story' also contextualises the Dora case, relating the case history to other patients and writings such as Emma from 'The Project' (1895) and 'The Psychogenesis of a Case of Homosexuality in a Woman' written in 1920. Lacan's reading of Freud's text is also at the centre of Ulrike Kadi's chapter: 'On the Signification of Dora's Father'. By focusing on a hitherto neglected parameter of the case history – the role of Dora's father – and furnishing the reader with biographical information on Philipp Bauer, Kadi provides a 'thick description' of the role of the father in psychoanalytic theory.

The final two chapters by Ilka Quindeau and Esther Hutfless both present readings of the Dora case in light of recent perspectives on hysteria, gender and sexuality. Indeed, Freud's text has attracted special attention by feminist criticism from the 1970s onwards. For Quindeau, it is the underlying theory of femininity which makes the Dora case so unsettling. In 'From Dora to Conchita: Recent Views on Gender and Sexuality in Psychoanalysis', she reads Dora as contesting heteronormativity, which is still one of the founding imperatives of our society in general and of psychoanalysis in particular. From the heteronormative assumptions which are at stake in the Dora case, Quindeau builds a bridge to the Austrian performer Conchita Wurst who, as a drag queen letting both masculinity and femininity exist side by side, won the Eurovision Song Contest in 2014, and discusses concepts of gender and sexuality which are beyond the binary regime. How to undermine the patriarchal, heteronormative and hegemonial order? This is also the overarching question in Esther Hutfless' contribution 'The Case of Dora – A Queer Perspective on Hysteria and Perversion'. Instead of delivering another re-reading of the Dora case, Hutfless analyses the vicissitudes of this text in the feminist discourse, and addresses key concepts such as perversion and hysteria. She argues for more profound debate between psychoanalysis and queer theory in order to keep the discussion on these major topics productive.

This volume would not have been possible without the support of the Sigmund Freud Foundation Vienna, the Sigmund-Freud-Stiftung in Frankfurt and the Vienna Municipal Department of Cultural Affairs. We would like to thank Richard Watts and Andrew Jenkins for their translation work, and Johanna Frei, Ulrike Kistner, Irene Popenberger, Gertrude Postl, Erika Umali and Kieryn Wurts-Hammond, for copy editing.

Daniela Finzi and Herman Westerink, August 2017

Narrative Strategies and Hermeneutic Desire: Constructions of a Case History

Daniela Finzi

One text and infinite effects

The 'Fragment of an Analysis of a Case of Hysteria' published in 1905 is Sigmund Freud's first independently published case history and his longest on a female patient, to whom he gave the alias 'Dora'. Together with the *Interpretation of Dreams* and the *Three Essays on the Theory of Sexuality*, the Dora case, which Freud originally intended to call 'Dream and Hysteria', constitutes the trilogy, as it were, of the 'founding texts' of psychoanalysis:[1] this term appears appropriate in so far as the writing of the text and treatment of the hysteria patient took place during the founding years of the new 'science of the unconscious' and the case history contains a number of key questions and landmarks in the formation of psychoanalytic theory. Since the publication of Felix Deutsch's 'A Footnote to Freud's "Fragment of an Analysis of a Case of Hysteria"'[2] in 1957 – at a time, that is, when the writing of psychoanalytic history was still governed by institutions and mostly centred on Freud – the case history has never ceased to appeal to subsequent generations and to elicit retorts. The 1970s and 1980s in particular saw a veritable deluge of psychoanalytic works. In a synopsis from 1986, Jerry L. Jennings classified this 'Dora Renaissance' according to the following topics: "Freud's (negative) counter transference"; "inadequate understanding of adolescent psychology"; "role of women in modern and Victorian society"; "biographical and historical information"; "concept of hysteria and the conversion process"; "literary and/or instructional value"; "homosexual currents not understood"; "neglect of transference interpretations"; "overly frank, ill-timed sexual interpretations";

---

[1] V. King, 'Fallgeschichte und Theorieentstehung. Produktivität und Grenzen der Erkenntnis in Freuds adoleszentem Fall Dora', in: G. Kimmerle (Ed.), *Zur Theorie der psychoanalytischen Fallgeschichte*. Tübingen: edition discord, 1998, pp. 45-83, p. 46.

[2] In this essay Deutsch revealed that he had treated Ida Bauer in 1922, who had since died, and could infer from her accounts that she had been Freud's former patient Dora. Another important essay for renewed interest in Dora was published five years later by Erik Erikson. F. Deutsch, 'A Footnote to Freud's "Fragment of an Analysis of a Case of Hysteria"', in: *Psychoanalytic Quarterly* 29 (1957), pp. 159-167; E. Erikson, 'Reality and Actuality: An Address', in: *Journal of the American Psychoanalytic Association* 10 (1962), pp. 451-474.

"misalliance of therapy goals".[3] The first emphatically literary piece focusing on the Dora case was published in 1974. Steven Marcus's powerful essay 'Freud and Dora: Story, History, Case History'[4] takes credit for opening the text to interpretations beyond the clinical, psychoanalytic discourse. As of the latter half of the 1970s and in the course of the 1980s, an increasing number of exponents of the women's movement and feminism began to discover this piece by Freud: as Claire Kahane wrote in her anthology *In Dora's Case. Freud – Hysteria – Feminism* first published together with Charles Bernheimer in 1985, "Dora is thus no longer read as merely a case history or a fragment of an analysis of hysteria but as an urtext in the history of woman, a fragment of an increasingly heightened critical debate about the meaning of sexual difference and its effects on the representations of feminine desire".[5]

Even today, another thirty years later, interest in Dora has not waned. In a later essay, Vera King, author of the monograph *Die Urszene der Psychoanalyse. Adoleszenz und Geschlechterspannung im Fall Dora* published in 1995, saw the reasons for the unfailing fascination of this Freud text in the fact that the Dora case deals with topics "that have been insufficiently understood or which have remained difficult in the 'modern' body of theory: gender tension and adolescence, topics and conflicts connected with female adolescence, the themes of the creative or creativity". The Dora case and the history of its reception, she observes, considers continuities and changes in gender relations; the case history has "thus become a paradigmatic point of reference for the resultant changes in theory formation".[6] In my opinion, a number of other factors must also be taken into account: the case history, entitled a 'Fragment', derives its particular appeal to a great extent from its form as both a fragment and a well-rounded whole, and from its explicit quality as a document of 'failure'. Even in the first pages of the preface, Freud uses such terms as "poor", "incomplete" and "shortcomings" to describe his case history.[7] Appealing implicitly to the credit of trust of his readers – to their willingness to believe him – he continues:

---

[3] Cf. J.L. Jennings: 'The Revival of Dora: Advances in Psychoanalytic Theory and Technique', in: *Journal of the American Psychoanalytical Association* 34 (1986), pp. 607–635, p. 621.
[4] S. Marcus, 'Freud and Dora: Story, History, Case History', in: C. Bernheimer & C. Kahane (Eds.), *In Dora's Case. Freud – Hysteria – Feminism*. Second Edition. New York: Columbia University Press 1990, pp. 56-91.
[5] C. Kahane, 'Introduction: Part Two', in: Bernheimer & Kahane, *In Dora's Case*, pp. 19-32, p. 31.
[6] V. King, ‚Fallgeschichte und Theorieentstehung', p. 45.
[7] Cf. S. Freud, 'A Fragment of an Analysis of a Case of Hysteria' (1905 [1901]), *SE* 7, pp. 3-122, p. 11ff. Freud's text is abbreviated to 'Dora' in the following.

"The treatment was not carried through to its appointed end, but was broken off at the patient's own wish when it had reached a certain point. At that time some of the problems of the case had not even been attacked and others had only been imperfectly elucidated; whereas, if the work had been continued, we should no doubt have obtained the fullest possible enlightenment upon every particular of the case. In the following pages, therefore, I can present only a fragment of an analysis."[8]

This supposedly curtailed offering holds immense potential: it makes no difference at all whether the fragment sets itself apart from the totality or whether it makes reference to it – the totality is always implicit. What Freud affords his readers is no different to what every narrative text offers: the possibility of putting oneself in the position of co-author. Whereas the formation of a "complementary story" is best observed at the end of the narrative text,[9] the reader of the Dora text is confronted from the outset with an 'unplanned' ending that offers room for alternative scenarios, as intended by the author. Whether intentional or not: this creates an author position in which the writing subject offers itself in a seductive act as an object of transference. Watching the author of this rhetorically brilliant piece 'fail' enables a reading experience rich in pleasure gain.[10]

The 'case history' of Dora as a "fine poetic conflict"[11]

While questions of gender relations and psychoanalytic theory formation constitute the starting point for the symposium 'Dora – Hysteria – Gender', from which this anthology is derived, the present contribution opts for a literary approach that stays close to the text with the aim of demonstrating the inherent literary potential of the Dora text and its proximity to literary methods and, in so doing, of arriving at new insights regarding its modes of functioning and effect. Special attention is thus given to the composition of this Freudian 'fragment' and its narrative strategies that are not only characteristic of this text, but which also give rise to constant attempts to induce interpretations and protest.[12] Note that the focus of my remarks is not, however, on the 'what',

---
[8] Ibid., pp. 12ff.
[9] Cf. F. K. Stanzel, 'Die Komplementärgeschichte. Entwurf einer leserorientierten Romantheorie', Stanzel: *Unterwegs. Erzähltheorie für Leser*. Göttingen: Vandenhoeck & Ruprecht 2002, pp. 307-328, p. 307ff.
[10] Cf. T. Anz, *Literatur und Lust. Glück und Unglück beim Lesen*. Munich: DTV, 2002.
[11] Freud, 'Fragment', p. 59.
[12] Cf. M. Bal, 'Lexicon for Cultural Analysis', in: A. Babka, D. Finzi & C. Ruthner (Eds.), *Die Lust an der Kultur/Theorie. Transdisziplinäre Interventionen. Für Wolfgang Müller-Funk*. Vienna: Turia+Kant 2012, pp. 49-81, p. 71.

but rather the 'how' of this account: in structuralist terms, the *discours* and not the *histoire* with all the different "sexual circuits".[13]

There were several reasons for the decision to tackle the Dora case with the instruments of literary analysis: first and foremost, it is due quite simply to the style of the text. An "amalgam of different genres including medical report, case history, psychoanalytic study, detective story or roman à clef",[14] it contains a myriad of literary and dramatic devices such as parallels, multilevel plots, flashbacks, reversals, variations, and so on. But the wide range of topics listed above and, to bring a term from literary reception aesthetics into play, the 'effects' of this psychoanalytic case history also suggest that we dissect it with literary instruments, i.e. that we understand it – similar to a fictional text – as a multi-layered entity and that we read it with a view to those passages of indeterminacy that are filled in the act of reading and thus initiate a kind of dialogue between the text and the reader.[15] What is more, the text itself invokes terms and devices from literature in various places: by making an initial distinction between the approach taken by a physician and by a writer, between "a contribution to the psychopathology of the neurosis"[16] and a novel, the categories to be discarded are in fact preserved and influence the reading. Dealing with Sigmund Freud as a modernist author, as it were, is justifiable in that he shares with this movement such methods as strategies of obscuration, a rejection of linear narrative, playing with subjective viewpoints and changing narrative perspectives, and extensive reader involvement.[17] Focusing on the dialogic, ambivalent and processual components of the Dora case history is not only useful with regard to literary questions, but rather demonstrates in all vehemence a specific fundamental feature found in both clinical and metapsychological Freud writings: they form a mixture of science and knowledge about the different scene of action and logic of the unconscious and operate with effects of transference and pleasure.[18]

---

[13] Cf. G. Genette, *Narrative Discourse. An Essay in Method*. Ithaca, NY: Cornell UP, 1995. Cf. on the question of "sexual circuits" J. Rose, 'Dora: "Fragment of an Analysis"', in: Bernheimer & Kahane, *In Dora's Case*, pp. 128-148, p. 131ff.

[14] M. Senarclens de Grancy, *Sprachbilder des Unbewussten. Die Rolle der Metaphorik bei Freud*. Gießen: Psycho-Sozial Verlag 2015, p. 164.

[15] W. Iser, *The Act of Reading. A Theory of Aesthetic Response*. Baltimore, MD: John Hopkins UP, 1991.

[16] Freud, 'Fragment', p. 9.

[17] Cf. Marcus, 'Freud and Dora', p. 69. Here we can only touch upon the complex and productive dynamic field between psychoanalysis and literature (literary studies) and the special importance played by literary texts in the development of Freud's theories. Freud used literary texts not only to illustrate theoretical concepts, but also as a medium for reflection on his own theory formation and as evidence for the scientific concepts.

[18] Cf. T. Anz, *Literatur und Lust*.

It should also be pointed out in this context that it is owed to the particular study of the case history as a genre that interest in the Dora case has increasingly shifted in recent years to epistemological questions as a result of coming to deal with the phenomenon of transference, whose structure and dynamics Freud describes in the critical commentary and postscript to the 'Fragment of an Analysis of a Case of Hysteria'.[19]

Indeed, case histories succeed like no other scientific medium in portraying the dynamics of cognitive and defence processes and in demonstrating the subjectivity of scientific work and the libidinous dynamics, demands and complications to which cognitive processes are subject. The Dora case in particular, in whose postscript Freud famously states his view on the phenomenon of transference in detail, presents Freud's involvement as a scientific subject in the cognitive process in what is in places a performative manner. The 'Fragment of an Analysis of a Case of Hysteria' – this much can be said from the outset – therefore demonstrates how profoundly the knowing subject, the object of knowledge, and the epistemological procedure are intertwined, and that a contrastive comparison of subject and world, research subject and research object is neither theoretically, nor empirically possible.[20]

For psychoanalysis, the case history medium is more than central and constitutive; as John Forrester noted, psychoanalysis – a world created almost wholly by actions of language that take place between analysand and analyst – involves "thinking in cases".[21] Indeed, epistemologically the 'case history' constitutes a special form of thinking. What is more, it is that special – textual – form of representation with which a life-story entrusted to the psychoanalyst is made public and scientifically relevant.[22] As in the historical and fictional narrative, temporality or the narrative link between different layers of time plays a key role in the psychoanalytic case history too.

---

[19] Cf. on increasing attention to rhetorical, narrative and media-specific forms and structures in the process of forming knowledge in the course of which case histories in particular became an object of research, S. Düwell & N. Pethes: 'Einleitung: Fall, Wissen, Repräsentation', in: S. Düwell & N. Pethes (Eds.), *Fall, Fallgeschichte, Fallstudie. Theorie und Geschichte einer Wissensform*. Frankfurt/New York: Campus 2014, pp. 9-33, p. 9.
[20] Cf. B. Nissen, 'Hat die Psychoanalyse die Struktur einer wissenschaftlichen Theorie?', in: *Psyche* 66,7 (2012), pp. 577-605.
[21] Cf. J. Forrester: *Thinking in cases*. John Wiley & Sons 2016. That the term 'case history' features not once in the writings of Freud, who wrote instead (of) medical histories [*Krankengeschichten*], can be explained by the fact that it only came into currency in German in the latter half of the 20th century. Cf. S. Düwell & N. Pethes: 'Einleitung: Fall, Wissen, Repräsentation', in: Düwell & Pethes, *Fall, Fallgeschichte, Fallstudie*, pp. 9-33, p. 11.
[22] Cf. on Freud's and Breuer's use of textual case histories to illustrate their methods in the context of controversy surrounding hypnosis in Vienna: A. Mayer, *Mikroskopie der Psyche. Die Anfänge der Psychoanalyse im Hypnose-Labor*. Göttingen: Wallstein 2002, p. 175ff.

When considering case histories in general and the Dora case in particular, account must be given to the fact that every individual undergoing psychoanalysis is subjected to various "stages of transformation" before appearing as a protagonist in the case history: this always involves multiple "rewritings of a life-story".[23] "Expecting immediacy from case histories arguably counts among the greatest, most persistent illusions of this genre".[24] While a case history without selecting material and without condensing content is a contradiction in terms,[25] this contradiction nevertheless does not release the author of a case history from his or her responsibility of depicting the 'how' of selection as transparently as possible and thereby enabling the reader to understand who is speaking when and how and with what intention. This question of how (and to what extent) the author Freud makes his decisions, omissions and constructions transparent, thus allowing the reader to distinguish between Dora's account and his own interpretation, will be explored later on; at this point let us note that every case history is always influenced a priori by multiple interpretations.

Structure and strategies

Divided by Freud into prefatory remarks, three sections, and a postscript,[26] the Dora case is based on what is both a simple and, on closer inspection, highly complex narrative structure consisting of a host of narrative levels and situations. In the manner of the narrator of a 'conventional' narrative, the first-person narrator builds up the suspense in the preface and framework story by announcing to his readers a world of "intimacies", "repressed wishes" and "secrets"[27] whose elucidation and particularly rendering in a public communication are for him a special challenge and duty to science. This framework story combines several different functions: as unsurprising as his intention may seem of installing the scientific subject and safeguarding the medical authority as a doctor, all the more salient is how firmly Freud establishes this undertaking by means of dialogue, giving consideration to the role of the reader. In an attempt to contextualise this case history in his own scientific biography, he also defines the requirements to be met by the "ideal reader" (Wolfgang Iser) – in his or her own interest: a satisfactory reading, he claims,

---

[23] Cf. P. Wegner, 'Die Fallgeschichte als Instrument psychoanalytischer Forschung', in: Kimmerle, *Zur Theorie der psychoanalytischen Fallgeschichte*, pp. 9-44, p. 18 ff.
[24] M. Wegener, 'Fälle, Ausfälle, Sündenfälle – Zu den Krankengeschichten Freud', in: Düwell & Pethes, *Fall, Fallgeschichte, Fallstudie*, pp. 169-194, p. 189.
[25] Cf. Wegner, 'Die Fallgeschichte als Instrument psychoanalytischer Forschung', p. 21.
[26] Part I is entitled 'The Clinical Picture' and is comparable in length to the parts on Dora's two 's ('II. The First Dream' and 'III. The Second Dream').
[27] Freud, 'Fragment', pp. 7ff.

is only possible for those familiar with the *Interpretation of Dreams*; readers of the *Studies on Hysteria*, in turn, are prepared for the fact that psychoanalytic technique has since been "completely revolutionized": as he says, in this new technique he "let[s] the patient himself choose the subject of the day's work". What appears at first sight to be a gesture of reserve is above all, to return to Freud's frequent metaphor of psychoanalysis as archaeology at that time, a clever prelude justifying his active construction in view of the aforementioned fragmentary nature of this case history: "I have restored what is missing, taking the best models known to me from other analyses; but, like a conscientious archaeologist, I have not omitted to mention in each case where the authentic parts end and my constructions begin".[28]

Just a few pages and the reader has been assigned a host of different roles, that this first-person narrator appears to have so effortlessly at his disposal: doctor, author, archaeologist, educator and taboo-breaker: "What is new has always aroused bewilderment and resistance".[29] The hysteria patient, described solely based on her gender and youth, remains anonymous and faceless, in contrast. Only after portraying the family circumstances in the first part ("I. The Clinical Picture") does the as yet nameless girl become a daughter and sister, with Freud – once again involving the reader – then proceeding to give her the "name Dora".[30] With regard to the arsenal of protagonists featuring in what he identifies as a "Victorian domestic drama", the aforementioned Steven Marcus also arrives at the following insight:

> "In fact, as the case history advances it becomes increasingly clear to the careful reader that Freud and not Dora has become the central character in the action. Freud the narrator does in the writing what Freud the first psychoanalyst appears to have done in actuality. We begin to sense that it is his story that is being written and not hers that is being retold. Instead of letting Dora appropriate her own story, Freud became the appropriator of it."[31]

It is exactly this question of appropriation that is spotlighted in numerous feminist writings on the Dora case: a question that can, however, only be answered exhaustively if we distance ourselves from a binary victim/perpetrator opposition and also ask the question as to Dora's complicity.

---

[28] Ibid., p. 12.
[29] Ibid., p. 11.
[30] Cf. regarding Freud's reasons for choosing this name his remarks in: *The Psychopathology of Everyday Life, SE* 6, p. 241ff.
[31] Marcus, 'Freud and Dora', pp. 56-91, p. 85.

In narratological terms, we are dealing with a "first-person narrative situation"[32] – that is to say, a first-person narrator who is himself a protagonist in the narrative and whose view of the narrated world hence comes 'from within'. In the canon of world literature, the first-person narrative situation is about as widespread and common as the 'authorial' one: the author in this case stands outside of the world he is narrating and is thus ascribed a certain omnipotence. The first-person narrative situation, in turn, is commonly attributed a certain 'naturalness'; its accepted merit is the relative ease with which the reader can identify with the first-person narrator: after all, "in the fictional world [he or she] takes up roughly the same position as that from which the first-person narrator experiences and narrates".[33] 'Experience and narration' – this not only denotes the particular situation of the first-person narrator, but also the central challenge of this narrative situation: the distance in time that lies between the experiencing and the narrating first person – between pre-narrative experience, on the one hand, and memory that retrospectively creates meaning, on the other – implies that the latter always has additional knowledge regarding the outcome of an action. On the other hand, it 'must' not reveal this knowledge (in the literary text) as every narrative thrives on suspense and delay.

A distinction can also be made in the Dora case between an experiencing and a narrating first person, the protagonist and the narrator of the story. In the sense of French literary theorist Philippe Lejeune, the identity of the protagonist, narrator and author also constitutes an "autobiographical pact".[34] The experiencing first person is deployed above all in the *in actu* passages concerning the two dreams and is directly involved in events, living through it in the moment: dialogue scenes and the present tense prevail here – that is to say, a seemingly direct 'showing' – embedded in passages of 'telling' written in retrospect. In the preface, in the parts describing the condition, and in the postscript, the focus is clearly on the narrating first person and thus on the act of narrating. This structure becomes increasingly complex as the narrator calls up a figure from the sub-plot, namely Dora's father, as a narrative figure presenting his view of the aetiology of the illness in indirect and direct speech.[35] On the other hand, the first-person narrator constantly oscillates between two different agents: on the one hand we see a narrating first person who talks about

---

[32] F. K. Stanzel, *A Theory of Narrative*. Cambridge: Cambridge University Press, 1979.
[33] Cf. C. Bode, *The Novel. An Introduction*. Chichester: Wiley-Blackwell, 2011, p. 120.
[34] P. Lejeune, *On Autobiography*. Minneapolis: University of Minnesota, 1989. The identity between author, narrator and protagonist explains my frequent use of the author's name instead of distinguishing consistently between author, narrating and experiencing first person.
[35] Freud, 'Fragment', pp. 85ff.

the conversations with Dora and about the progress of therapy in late autumn of 1900, thus suggesting a closeness in time to the experiencing first person, while on the other there is the narrative agent who comments on the case from the time – or rather times[36] – of writing, adding theoretical annotations and contextualising the case in Freud's scientific biography. Just as Freud mingled the particular case history with previously gained insights and premises in the course of analysis, so too did he in the subsequent process of writing up – and it is not always possible to make a clear-cut distinction from case to case. Special emphasis should also be given to the fact that the particular case is repeatedly supplemented and explained by means of more general psychoanalytic knowledge in the Dora case – "[I]t is a rule of psycho-analytic technique that (…)",[37] – or that, in some cases, the details of the specific case are supplanted by more general positions.

It is also the narrating first person who engages in extremely active contact with the reader by regularly informing him or her about the next steps and methodological considerations and addressing any expectations.[38] Equally, it is also pointed out whenever the narrator begins to "construct", filing in any "gaps", and, by so doing, taking what might be referred to as steps of fictionalisation:[39] not only does he mention the lack of session notes and emphasise the intentional change in the "order in which the explanations are given (…) for the sake of presenting the case in a more connected form". Incompleteness and thus a potential for fictionalisation also result from the fact that the narrator, as he concedes in his prefatory remarks, "(has) not reproduced the process of interpretation to which the patient's associations and communications had to be subjected, but only the results of that process". He goes on to observe that his recollection of "the order in which (…) conclusions were reached" was not always equally reliable.[40] Implicitly, the narrator or Freud also concedes that his reconstruction of a key scene is based on his own imagination: "If I may suppose that the scene of the kiss took place in this way (…)".[41] Not only is the reader regularly informed about these constructions, about the processes of guessing and filling that the doctor must perform – the transitions from

---
[36] After treatment was broken off, Freud wrote up the case history in January 1901, and revised the paper before its publication 1905.
[37] Ibid., p. 39.
[38] Cf. also M. Krause, 'Seelensucher'. Freuds "Bruchstück einer Hysterie-Analyse" als Versuchsanordnung zwischen Literatur und Wissenschaft', in: M. Bies & M. Gamper (Eds.), *"Es ist ein Laboratorium für Worte". Experiment und Literatur III: 1890-2010.* Göttingen: Wallstein 2011, pp. 72-95, p. 85.
[39] See also, S. Freud, 'Constructions in Analysis' (1937), *SE* 23, pp. 255-269.
[40] Freud, 'Fragment', p. 95.
[41] Ibid., p. 31.

suspicion to certainty and from assumption to confirmation are also made quite clear.[42] Equally, Freud makes no secret of the fact that his approach is based on theoretical presuppositions and the concomitant 'obligations' and possible consequences: "If, therefore, the trauma theory is not to be abandoned, (...)".[43]

Case histories are always written with the aim of signalling a further development of theory – and are thus intentional texts. Once again, Freud also shares his intentions with the reader: his aim, as he sets forth on the very first page, is to show "that the causes of hysterical disorders are to be found in the intimacies of the patients' psycho-sexual life, and that hysterical symptoms are the expression of their most secret and repressed wishes";[44] and he aims to show "how dream-interpretation is woven into the history of a treatment and how it can become the means of filling in amnesias and elucidating symptoms".[45] In my opinion it is not the intentionality of the text itself that creates a need for explanation, given that it is indicated and conceded in the establishing remarks at the beginning and end – instead, it is the extent and effects of this intentionality that necessitate closer consideration. For the reader, one particular effect of the latter is the fact that the text is dominated by a legitimising tone, effacing all trace of "evenly-suspended attention". In order to 'understand' Freud's endeavours to ensure 'applicability',[46] it is worthwhile considering not only the "intertextual" context, as it is known in literary studies, (i.e. the relationship between the text and other texts), but also the "extratextual" context (i.e. the "relationship of a text to non-textual circumstances")[47] and to contextualise the Dora case in the history of the nascent psychoanalytic movement and to interpret it as a strategic intervention.

At the date of writing up the case history in January 1901, and at the date of revising in 1905, prior to going to press, *The Interpretation of Dreams* was still a long way away from its subsequent status as the world's most famous psychoanalytic publication and 'book of the century'. The first edition had sold a mere six hundred copies; as Freud notes in the preface to the Dora case, he had met with only "an inadequate degree of comprehension" among other specialists.[48] The letters to Wilhelm Fliess in autumn 1899, following publication

---

[42] Ibid., p. 94, p. 99.
[43] Ibid., p. 27.
[44] Ibid., pp. 8ff.
[45] Ibid., p. 10.
[46] Ibid., p. 128, p. 170.
[47] L. Danneberg, 'Kontext', in: H. Fricke (Ed.), *Reallexikon der deutschen Literaturwissenschaft*. 2nd vol., H – O. 3rd, revised ed. Berlin et al.: de Gruyter 2000, pp. 333-336, p. 333.
[48] Freud, 'Fragment', p. 10.

of the book, testify to Freud's perception of the reception of the *Interpretation of Dreams* and his disappointment at the perceived ignorance or lack of a positive response. Meanwhile, although Freud's own view of the early academic isolation of psychoanalysis and the reserved reception of *The Interpretation of Dreams* has been refuted, Freud must nevertheless, as he observes in his letters to Fliess, have felt the early years up to 1905 to be a "splendid isolation".[49]

Thanks to these letters from Freud to Fliess we also know that he let his correspondent know as early as 14 October 1900 that his new patient was "a case that has smoothly opened to the existing collection of picklocks".[50] From a very early point in the analysis, Freud was thus interested in the soundness and potential evidential value of the case – which, in other words, means that the interpretation to be developed in the course of treatment was substantially marked by certain presuppositions. Certainly, Freud's words to Fliess were always charged with the wish to impress him, the other man – but even without any knowledge of this note, one cannot help but sense while reading Dora's case history that he constructed the account towards a preconceived outcome or result, at least in terms of the textual representation. What we have here are not merely partial reading impressions, but a phenomenon of circularity familiar from *The Interpretation of Dreams*. When Freud recounts his dreams, he arranges them in such a way that the subsequent interpretation is as if tailor-made – which is not surprising given that narrative and interpretation come from one and the same source.[51]

Hermeneutic circle, narrative coherence, lack of complicity

As a humanistic discipline, psychoanalysis is afflicted by the same paradox known as the 'hermeneutic circle', whereby that which is to be understood must already have been understood beforehand: meaning is always created by conflating a sign – of a dream, a patient's statement – with existing or supposed

---

[49] Cf. Letter 244 of 7 May 1900 to Fliess, in: *The Complete Letters of Sigmund Freud to Wilhelm Fliess. 1887–1904*. J.M. Masson (Ed.). Cambridge, MA: The Belknap Press of Harvard University Press, 1985, p. 412. Cf. on the reception of *The Interpretation of Dreams* N. Kiell, *Freud without hindsight. Reviews of His Work* (1893–1939). Madison, CT: International Universities Press 1988, pp. 87-91; p. 89: "(…) I found 21 substantial reviews published between 1899 and 1902, with another 20 between 1903 and 1915. (…) An additional 24 reviews came out between 1916 and 1975, as well as countless exegeses." Cf. also T. Elliger: 'Sigmund Freuds "splendid isolation". Materialien zur Kritik der psychoanalytischen Geschichtsschreibung', in: *Psyche* 44 (1990), pp. 612-627.

[50] Cf. letter 255, 14/10/1900, in: *The Complete Letters of Sigmund Freud to Wilhelm Fliess. 1887–1904*, p. 427.

[51] J. Le Rider, 'Freud. Schreiben, Lesen und Heilen', in: Babka, Finzi & Ruthner, *Die Lust an der Kultur/Theorie*, pp. 190-203, p. 193.

knowledge about the world, reality and theory. The term 'hermeneutic desire' in the title of this paper emphasises this fact: if, thanks to psychoanalysis, we can develop an understanding of the fact that all categories created in the process of scientific work and communication are equally structured by desire, no one better than Freud himself informs us of this 'pleasure in generating knowledge'. Viewed from this perspective, Freud's interpretation of the case study reveals more about his own hermeneutic desire – that is, to demonstrate the validity of psychosexual aetiology – than about what Dora really experienced and suffered. Reacting to the suggestion that her mother's jewel-case from the first dream could be interpreted as a symbol for the female genitalia, for example, Dora noted: "I knew you would say that". Whereupon Freud cleverly incorporated her rebuke into the narrative that he wanted to have confirmed: "That is to say, you knew that it *was* so".[52], adding in a footnote: "A very common way of putting aside a piece of knowledge that emerges from the repressed". But perhaps this passage can also be seen as a sign that Dora must very soon have discovered which kind of stories satisfied him and won Freud over?[53]

Freud's appropriation of Dora's statements brings us to a *hermeneutics of suspicion* inherent in psychoanalysis that transcends this case history: there is no disputing that with psychoanalysis Sigmund Freud developed a narrative model which enabled new narratives of identity and new formats of self-description. One of their characteristic traits is that they can no longer be clearly classified as being on one side of the distinction between normality and perversion – an unquestionably revolutionary and emancipatory step compared with hitherto predominant notions of health and sickness that are, incidentally, all cultural constructions and discursive posits. Nevertheless, Freud's refusal to make a qualitative distinction between normality and pathology and his idea that both are immediately contiguous led to an "epistemology of suspicion" towards any kind of ordinary behaviour.[54] In this respect, the mode of interpretation of Freud's psychoanalysis might be referred to as symptomatic; the aim is always to discover hidden meanings, hidden sense.[55]

In terms of the Dora case history, this would mean that, in view of Freud's enormous presuppositions described above, little or no space remains for her desire and her rebellion in that while Dora is able to speak and articulate 'words

---

[52] Freud, 'Fragment', p. 69.
[53] J. Forrester & L. Appignanesi, *Freud's Women*. London: Weidenfeld and Nicolson, 1992, p. 150.
[54] Cf. E. Illouz, *Saving the Modern Soul. Therapy, Emotions, and the Culture of Self-Help*. Berkeley, CA: University of California Press, 2008, p. 4.
[55] Admittedly, my remarks about Freud's supposed intentions also corresponded to a symptomatic reading.

of protest', that were indeed heard – as evidenced in Freud's account, that abounds with examples illustrating Dora's objections – they were not, however, interpreted or reframed. A "most emphatic negative"[56] can be cited as evidence of his line of argumentation: Dora's 'No' must be due to repression – with this presupposition "the first evidence soon begins to appear that in such a case 'No' signifies the desired 'Yes'".[57]

Let us return from symptomatic reading to the narratological perspective: where the 'genre' of the case history in itself refers to narrative theory, its subject – the narrative – refers to a central mode in psychoanalysis: indeed, narrating plays a pre-eminent role in psychoanalytic treatment, also known as the 'talking cure'. Paul Ricœur described the goal of this omnipresent cultural technique as follows in *Time and Narrative*: "to substitute for the bits and pieces of stories that are unintelligible as well as unbearable (…) a coherent and acceptable story, in which the analysand can recognize his or her self-constancy".[58] The ideal notion of coherence is also a central theme in the Dora case history, and one which defines the first few pages. In one passage that is once again dedicated to establishing a trusting, sound relationship with the reader, we read: "If I were to begin by giving a full and consistent case history, it would place the reader in a very different situation from that of the medical observer".[59] With the same firmness with which he rejects the "smooth and precise histories in cases of hysteria" familiar from other authors as questionable, he notes "The patients' inability to give an ordered history of their life in so far as it coincides with the history of their illness".[60] The patients' narrative, to paraphrase Freud with narratological terms, is "unreliable"[61] as it is imperfect; the motives given for this include deliberate reserve or dishonesty; unconscious dishonesty and amnesias. Here we can make out an aim of the treatment: ultimately, to survey "an intelligible, consistent, and unbroken case history".[62] That this endeavour comes at the expense of the sublimation wishes, needs and fantasies of the Dora figure comes as no real surprise.

---

[56] Freud, 'Fragment', p. 58.
[57] Ibid., p. 59. Cf. also King, 'Fallgeschichte und Theorieentstehung', p. 59.
[58] P. Ricœur, *Time and Narrative*. Vol. III: Narrated Time. Chicago: University of Chicago Press, 1998, p. 247.
[59] Freud, 'Fragment', p. 16.
[60] Ibid., p. 95.
[61] Cf. on the 'unreliable narrator' W. C. Booth, *The Rhetoric of Fiction*. Chicago: University of Chicago Press, 1961.
[62] Freud, 'Fragment', p. 18. Cf. also on this interpretation of attempts at coherence Marcus Krause, who likens Freud's textual interventions to the interventions of the unconscious in the dream, Krause, 'Seelensucher', p. 12.

The criterion cited by Ricœur, in contrast – the (re)cognition of self-constancy – does not appear to feature explicitly in Freud's phrasing; and of course, we can interpret Dora's termination of treatment as showing that the narrative uncovered or constructed by Freud and his normative male expectations of female sexual response did not tally with her story or her self-constancy. Only after breaking off treatment – breaking free of the narrative imposed on her by Freud – as we learn in the postscript, does Dora succeed in taking that critical step that, in my opinion, Freud was unwilling to support fully during treatment:[63] at a meeting with the Ks

> "she made it up with them, she took her revenge on them, and she brought her own business to a satisfactory conclusion. To the wife she said: 'I know you have an affair with my father'; and the other did not deny it. From the husband she drew an admission of the scene by the lake which he had disputed, and brought the news of her vindication home to her father."[64]

What Dora accomplished here is more than remarkable and in my opinion provides us with one of the 'picklocks' for a deeper understanding of her case history: I am referring to the insult that grows out of the exchange[65] to which Dora was subject. In the words of feminist anthropologist Gayle Rubin, "'exchange of women' [is] a shorthand for expressing that the social relations of a kinship system specify that men have certain rights in their female kin, and that women do not have the same rights either to themselves or to their male kin".[66]

How does Freud behave in this matter? Although he undoubtedly lent Dora his ear and his credence that her father was having an affair with Mrs K. and that she, his own daughter, had been handed over to Mr K. in exchange; and although Freud did not fulfil the implicit task set by Dora's father,[67] he nevertheless erred

---

[63] Although it must be said at this point in Freud's defence that he had assumed a lengthier duration of treatment and that this consolidation may have been part of his therapeutic goals.
[64] Freud, 'Fragment', p. 121.
[65] Cf. C. Lévi-Strauss, *The Elementary Structures of Kinship*. London: Eyre & Spottiswoode, 1969.
[66] G. Rubin, 'The Traffic in Women: Notes on the Political Economy of Sex', in: R.R. Reiter, *Toward an anthropology of women*. New York: Monthly Review Press, 1975, pp. 157-210, p. 177.
[67] The task indicated in the case history is: "Please try and bring her to reason." Freud, 'Fragment', p. 26. Behind this was a request for Freud to stop Dora demanding that her father break off contact with Mrs K.

in accusing her of being partly to blame for the affair between the father and Mrs K., appearing interested in neither causality nor emotional dependencies. Worse still, in the course of the narrative, his supposed advocacy of objectivity in judging the incidents turn into efforts above all of finding Dora guilty of vindictiveness and of masturbation. I do not deny Freud's intention of curing the young patient, of affording her – as he writes of his patients in the *Studies on Hysteria* – "help and improvement", and of helping her achieve a "mental life that has been restored to health"[68]. Yet today we recognise that Ida Bauer, who passed the time with "attending lectures for women" and "more or less serious studies",[69] would quite obviously have claimed her place in her social, patriarchal environment. The support that she would have needed in order to resist the demands and contradictions required of her by family and society was not afforded her by her doctor. This omission also plays a part, unconsciously, in the ambivalent and emotionally charged relationship between the author and his readers.

* * *

It is true that as readers we can only experience the Dora figure as Freud portrayed her: as a memory of her words that he could and wanted to recall, as traces of her statements that tallied with his 'theory novel'. Yet a careful reading not only reveals all those places in which Freud indicates his constructions and at least gives the reader the opportunity to undertake his or her own reconstruction of the events discussed. It also shows that the text actually does contain traces of Dora's involvements that did not correspond to Freud's heteronormative focus. Dora's tender unconscious affections for Mrs K. were certainly noted by Freud and were covered in the case history, if not in the treatment. In order to make Dora a "complete figure" and to gain an insight into her thoughts, it may be necessary to switch media. Thus it is probably no coincidence that Hélène Cixous not only wrote the study *La jeune née*, but also a play entitled *Portrait de Dora* in 1975; four years before Anthony McCall and Claire Pajaczkowska presented *Sigmund Freud's Dora*, a masterpiece of feminist film, as a *Case of Mistaken Identity*. Narrative researchers agree with Käthe Hamburger that only in fiction is it possible to look inside other people's thoughts and thus preserve a sense of "first-person originality".[70]

---

[68] S. Freud, 'The Psychotherapy of Hysteria', in: J. Breuer & S. Freud, *Studies on Hysteria* (1895), *SE* 2, pp. 253-305, p. 305.
[69] Freud, 'Fragment', p. 101.
[70] Cf. M. Fludernik, *Erzähltheorie. Eine Einführung*. Darmstadt: WGB, 2010, p. 86.

The Analytic Denial of Freud's Struggle with the Understanding of Dora: Simplifying the Oedipus Complex and the Process of its Adoption

Rachel B. Blass

The Oedipal reading of Dora

The most common critique of Freud's case study of Dora is that in this study Freud applied a limited Oedipal model, which stood in the way of more nuanced understanding of her dynamics, and more generally of the dynamics of an adolescent girl.

Erikson in the first actual critique of the case points to Freud's undivided concern with "genetic truth" and the better understanding of the unconscious, to the neglect of "historical truth", which is of utmost importance for a developing adolescent such as Dora. Furthermore, for Erikson, Freud's "genetic truth" centered on "psychosexual and Oedipal" formulations.[1] Freud's assignment to the father of the role of the "hoped-for protector of his daughter's inviolacy" is seen to be a somewhat surprising exception to Freud's general tendency to limit the girl's concerns to libidinal wishes to be seduced by the father, the need to repress such wishes, and the desire to find appropriate substitutes for him. Following Erikson, others have criticized Freud's inappropriate treatment of adolescent transference[2] and his overwhelming of the adolescent ego with adult Oedipal interpretations.[3]

In the mid-1970s a renewed interest in technique led to more detailed analyses of Freud's interactions with Dora.[4] The view that Freud adhered to a positive Oedipal model, however, remained constant. Thus, it was argued, Freud considered Dora's transference to be founded on early real and fantasied

---

[1] E. H. Erikson, 'Reality and actuality', in: *Journal of the American Psychoanalytic Association* 10 (1962), pp. 451-474, p. 462.
[2] C. Adatto, 'On the metamorphosis from adolescence into adulthood', in: *Journal of the American Psychoanalytic Association* 14 (1966), pp.485-509.
[3] *See*, Schlesinger,in: J. Lindon, 'A psychoanalytic view of the family', in: *The Psychoanalytic forum* 3 (1969), pp.11-65; P. Blos, 'The epigenesis of the adult neurosis', in: *The Psychoanalytic Study of the Child* 27 (1972), pp.106-135.
[4] R. Langs, 'The misalliance dimension in Freud's case histories', in: *The International Journal of Psychoanalysis* 5 (1976), pp.301-317; N. Muslin & M. M. Gill, 'Transference in the Dora case', in: *Journal of the American Psychoanalytic Association* 26 (1978), pp. 311-328.

experiences with *parental* figures.⁵ Some of the studies of Dora's transference turn our attention to two new questions: one pertains to the place of the countertransference. Freud's unawareness of both his libidinal, Oedipal strivings in relation to his young patient and his negative countertransference arising especially in response to her rejection of these strivings receive extensive notice.⁶ The second question that arises has to do with the role of the mother in the transference and especially Freud's *neglect* of this important component of the Oedipal constellation.⁷

Freud's Oedipal understandings of Dora have also been counterposed to various forms of pre-Oedipal and early Oedipal understandings.⁸ Blos, for example, speaks of Freud's "pursuing with single-minded pertinacity the positive Oedipal theme"⁹ throughout Dora's analysis, a pursuit which resulted in the de-emphasis of the importance of the pre-Oedipal issues of adolescence. In a similar vein Krohn and Krohn inform us that "Freud conceptualized Dora's pathology as representing primarily positive Oedipal conflicts".¹⁰ Here it is the understanding of Dora in terms of her phallic-Oedipal constellation¹¹ that is purportedly neglected.

Other reviews of Freud's analysis of Dora have come from feminist circles.¹² Freud's purported focus on Oedipal fantasy usually is introduced in the context of a critique of his obliviousness to the actuality of Dora's seduction. Freud's understanding of Dora in terms of Oedipal fantasy is viewed as the product of his mistaken abandonment of his early theories which ascribed to incest and actual seduction the most prominent pathogenic role.

In a more general way, however, most reviews of the Dora case see in it a sharp break, in the main a positive one, from his earlier theory of seduction. Krohn and Krohn reflect the prevalent sentiment in their description of Dora's case as the first to be presented in the "psychoanalytic phase as opposed to the pre-

---

⁵ M. Kanzer & J. Glenn (Eds.), *Freud and His Patients.* New York: Aronson 1980, chaps. 1 to 5.
⁶ E.g. J. Glenn, 'Freud's adolescent patients', in: ibid., pp. 23-47; I. Bernstein, 'Integrative summary: On the reviewings of the Dora case', in: ibid., pp. 83-91.
⁷ E.g. K. Lewin, 'Dora revisited', in: *The Psychoanalytic Review* 60 (1973), pp. 519-532.
⁸ P. Blos, *The Adolescent Passage.* New York: International University Press, 1979; A. Krohn & J. Krohn, 'The nature of the Oedipus complex in the Dora case', in: *Journal of the American Psychoanalytic Association* 30 (1982), pp. 555-578; G. Kohon, 'Reflections on Dora', in: *The International Journal of Psychoanalysis* 65 (1984), pp. 73-84.
⁹ Blos, *The Adolescent Passage*, p. 488.
¹⁰ Krohn & Krohn, 'The nature of the Oedipus complex in the Dora case', p. 558.
¹¹ H. Nagera, *Female Sexuality and the Oedipus Complex.* New York: Aronson, 1975.
¹² See, C. Bernheimer & C. Kahane (Eds.), *In Dora's Case: Freud, Hysteria, Feminism.* New York: Columbia University Press, 1985.

analytic phase of his work".[13] Likewise, the historian Peter Gay discussed the Dora case under the heading of "A Problematic Debut".[14] Slipp[15] and Spiegel[16] pointed to Freud's overemphasis of fantasy to the neglect of interpersonal factors and actual seduction. They tie these to Freud's recognition of the failure of his seduction theory. Accordingly, examinations from the historical perspective tend to be directed toward the study of the relationship between the Oedipal framework Freud worked with in Dora's analysis and those that evolved in the course of the following 100 years.

The mistake

The problem with these assessments of Freud's Oedipal interpretations of Dora – both the positive and negative assessments – is that they neglect the reality of Freud's understanding of Dora. It's not that his Oedipal interpretations were better or worse than presented. He simply did not offer Oedipal interpretations. I made this point some 25 years ago in a paper entitled 'Did Dora have an Oedipus complex?', which had been translated into German and appeared as 'Hatte Dora einen Ödipuskomplex?', published in the *Jahrbuch der Psychoanalyse* in 1994.[17] The answer to the question of the title is simply 'no'. At the time of Dora's analysis, as well as at the time of its publication approximately five years later, Freud's ideas concerning the Oedipal dynamics and their role in normal and pathological development had not reached the consolidation ascribed to them in each and every one of the later studies of the case.

In what follows I will briefly illustrate this. I will show, with the help of a few examples, that Freud's understanding of Dora was not at all Oedipal. This raises the interesting question of *how* Freud's question could have been so grossly misread. I will not go into this question, which I discussed in my earlier work. Instead I will focus on the consequences of this misreading and its possible causes. I will argue that by making Dora an Oedipal case Freud's Oedipal model and the process of its adoption is simplified. It's as though Oedipal thinking is the natural or obvious alternative to Freud's earlier ideas on trauma and seduction and once those were put aside it we have 'Oedipus'. The fact of the matter is that the Oedipal complex is more complex, and not so readily adoptable. I go

---

[13] Krohn & Krohn, 'The Nature of the Oedipus complex in the Dora case', p. 556.
[14] P. Gay, *Freud: A Life for Our Time*. New York: Norton 1988.
[15] S. Slipp, 'Interpersonal factors in hysteria', in: *Journal of the American Psychoanalytic Association* 5 (1977), pp. 359-376.
[16] R. Spiegel, 'Freud and the women in his world', in: *Journal of the American Psychoanalytic Association*. 5 (1977), pp. 377-402.
[17] R.B. Blass, 'Hatte Dora einen Ödipuskomplex?', in: *Jahrbuch der Psychoanalyse* 32 (1994), pp. 74-111.

on to suggest that the analytic assumption that Freud held his Oedipal model already at the time of 'Dora' conceals some of the difficulties involved in the adoption of the Oedipus complex. In my earlier work, I emphasized one of these difficulties. Today I would like to outline also some additional ones. These difficulties relate to determining the origins of the complex and of guilt and the basic meaning and nature of sexuality and its perverse expressions. They also pertain to the dangers experienced in committing to a new analytic theory. By acknowledging Freud's struggle with his ideas that we can come to better appreciation of their significance.

The non-Oedipal nature of Freud's understanding of Dora

Before turning to the examples of the non-Oedipal nature of Freud's understanding I think it's helpful to take a look at what Freud says about his understanding. This is how he opens the Dora text, under the heading of 'Prefatory remarks':

> "In 1895 and 1896 I put forward certain views upon the pathogenesis of hysterical symptoms and upon the mental processes occurring in hysteria. Since that time several years have passed. In now proposing, therefore, to substantiate those views by giving a detailed report of the history of a case and its treatment, I cannot avoid making a few introductory remarks (…)."[18]

In other words Freud opens the text by stating in no uncertain terms that this case history is being presented to substantiate the views on hysteria that he put forth in 1895 and 1896. What he refers to here are his *Studies on Hysteria*[19] and other early papers on hysteria[20] in which Freud famously brings forth his seduction/trauma theory understandings of hysteria. He explicitly states that he is presenting Dora to validate non-Oedipal models. In fact, he speaks as though no significant developments have taken place; here is yet another case confirming his models, which remain those that he put forth about a decade earlier.

I don't think this is an accurate description on Freud's part. What he describes doesn't confirm those early models exactly, but they also do not refer to an Oedipal model. Here are some examples of why not:

---

[18] S. Freud, 'Fragment of an Analysis of a Case of Hysteria' (1905), *SE* 7, pp. 3-122, p. 7.
[19] J. Breuer & S. Freud, *Studies on Hysteria* (1895), *SE* 2.
[20] E.g., S. Freud, 'The Aetiology of Hysteria' (1896), *SE* 3. pp. 189-221.

Psychic trauma: Freud's initial explanation of Dora's pathology is in line with his trauma theory proposed in *Studies on Hysteria*. As Freud explains, "[t]he experience with Herr K. – his making love to her and the insult to her honour which was involved – seems to provide in Dora's case the psychical trauma which Breuer and I declared long ago to be the indispensable prerequisite for the production of a hysterical disorder."[21]

In accordance with this theory, the trauma which occurred when Dora was 16 years old would lead to pathology only if it came into association with an earlier repressed trauma. Thus, in Dora's case, Freud proceeds to seek out the earlier trauma and comes up with Herr K.'s kiss in the doorway when Dora was but 14 years old.

Repressed love for the seducer: Later Freud suggests that what is ultimately responsible for Dora's symptoms are her forbidden longings for him, the symptoms being symbolic expressions of these longings and libidinal wishes. This proposition in many ways resembles Freud's formulation of hysteria as the result of the repression of "incompatible ideas".[22]

The role of the father: At some point in the text Freud refers to the necessary involvement of sexual fantasy in hysteria, but strikingly when Freud first introduces this idea he regards the fact that in Dora's case the fantasy is tied to the father is accidental, not necessary. Freud explains that it was the "wearisome monotony" with which Dora kept repeating her complaints against her father that led Freud to suspect that her symptoms "might have some meaning in connection with her father".[23] The conjunction of the chance connection with the father and Freud's 'rule' of the necessary involvement of sexual fantasy is the only reason presented here for Freud's later interest in pursuing Dora's sexual-affectionate ties with her father.

When he does so later on in the text Freud suggests that Dora's intense love of her father, which was seen to be responsible for several of her symptoms is itself a "reactive symptom", arising in attempts to suppress intense feelings of love for her seducer, Herr K. That is, Freud proposes that Dora "summon[ed] up her infantile affection for her father and (…) exaggerate[d] it, in order to protect herself against the feelings of love which were constantly pressing forward into consciousness".[24] Here the primary love object is clearly Herr K, not the father. In fact, when Freud is later concerned with his failure to take note of

---

[21] Freud, 'Fragment', p. 7.
[22] E.g., the cases of Lucy R. and Elisabeth von R. in the *Studies on Hysteria*.
[23] Ibid., p. 46.
[24] Ibid., p. 58.

the transference he's wondering about transference tied to Dora's relationship with Herr K, not "father transference" as often thought.[25] Nevertheless, in this context Freud does speak of a universal bond between father and daughter, mentioning the existence of a "sexual attraction (…) felt between parents and children" which typically appears at an early age and which has been poetically described in the "legend of Oedipus".[26] It is very important to take note, however, that counter to what he posits in his Oedipal model Freud contends that when this attraction to the parent persists past infancy in the form of an underlying "sexual inclination", pathology is implicated, this later "sexual inclination" being seen as a manifestation of "a fixation of this rudimentary feeling of love".[27]

Masturbation and fixation: Later still Freud arrives at the conclusion that it was Dora's masturbatory practices that were responsible for her neurosis. He informs Dora that "she was now on the way to finding an answer to her own question of why it was that precisely she had fallen ill – by confessing that she had masturbated, probably in childhood."[28]

Masturbation is relevant because the hysteric both repudiates masturbation and remains fixated to it and thus produces symptoms that "substitute for masturbatory satisfaction".[29] Later Freud goes on to tie these ideas together with his thoughts on the seducer: "(…) if Dora felt unable to yield to her love for the man [who was her tempter, RBB], if in the end she repressed that love instead of surrendering to it, there was no factor upon which her decision depended more directly than upon her premature sexual enjoyment and its consequence – her bed-wetting, her catarrh, and her disgust."[30]

Freud's writing here is not completely clear, but it would seem that his thinking is that this moral repudiation of masturbation may become intimately associated with a sense of disgust with oneself and more specifically with one's genitals. This disgust is projected onto the sexuality of the seducer and reinforces the tendency to reject him.[31]

If one follows Freud's propositions concerning Dora, it becomes immediately apparent that an Oedipal constellation is not what lies at the heart of Dora's hysteria, nor does it lie at the heart of Freud's ideas on pathology in general. The

---

[25] Muslin & Gill, 'Transference in the Dora case', p. 317.
[26] Freud, 'Fragment', p. 56.
[27] Ibid.
[28] Ibid., p. 76.
[29] Ibid., p. 79.
[30] Ibid., p. 87.
[31] See, ibid., p. 84.

Oedipal drama is mentioned, but at this point Freud considers the unconscious retention of the infantile sexual affection for the father to be a manifestation of pathology, not a feature of normal development; and the retention of this sexual force is, on the whole, associated with an actual event – masturbation or the trauma of seduction. More importantly, the emergence of the love for the father is considered to be secondary feature. It is primarily presented as a defensive manoeuvre aimed at the repression of the primary conflict which is experienced in relation to the seducer. Complicated relations with one's father are clearly not presented as a prerequisite of neurosis. Thus both in terms of the quantitative force and of the qualitative content it is apparent that Freud has not yet arrived at an Oedipal formulation. This is further attested to by Freud's explicit statements that in Dora's case he was primarily interested in providing evidence that would 'substantiate' his views put forth in 1895 and 1896.

Overlooked difficulties and the simplification of the Oedipus complex

I will now briefly discuss three kinds of difficulties with Freud's Oedipal model that get overlooked by wrongly presenting Dora as an instance of Freud's application of that model. That is, by presenting Dora as an Oedipal case, the analytic community expresses the view that the adoption of this model was straightforward, a natural and obvious consequence of the abandonment of his earlier models and supported by Freud's Oedipal insights in the course of his self-analysis. This is not the case. The adoption of the Oedipal model is not simple and took Freud many years of hard work and difficult struggles, both personal and conceptual.

The first of the overlooked difficulties has to do with *the danger in committing to any new theory*, following the abandonment of his earlier ones. In a series of papers, I've closely studied Freud's early theories, how Freud confirmed them and what led to their abandonment. The picture that emerged was quite different than the official ones (as well as of the official critiques, e.g., the feminist ones) and specifically the abandonment was much more painful and problematic then we have been led to believe, including at times by Freud himself. In terms of the issues at hand what is most important is that the problems involved were of a kind that made Freud hesitant to adopt any new theory. I explain:

In discussing Freud's abandonment of his early theories, often referred to (wrongly) as his 'seduction theory' (Freud never used that term), his letter to Fliess of September 21, 1897 is commonly adduced. There he lists four reasons for leaving the theories he held at that time: his failure to bring a single case to conclusion; the unlikelihood that there exists such a high incidence of seductive fathers; the theoretical impossibility of distinguishing between actuality and affectively cathected fantasy; and the recognition that the unconscious can never be fully tamed by consciousness and hence treatment could never be complete. But from the study of Freud's writings[32] it is quite clear that he was aware of these arguments all along and felt that he had adequately responded to them. It is also clear that the discovery of his own Oedipal dynamics did not lead him to conclude that his patient's reports were expressions of phantasy. He had maintained for some time that he had Oedipal phantasies and hysteria was the result of seduction. Rather what Freud gradually came to recognize – albeit latently – was the seductive effect of his theories; that in putting forth his seduction theory he played a very seductive role in relation to his patients, procuring from them reports that would support his ideas on seduction. In other words, confrontation with his own Oedipal fantasies which included seductive fantasies involving the 'daughter' led Freud unconsciously to suspect the effect these fantasies had on his theory, his method, and his relationship with his young female patients. He saw that the patients' reports of their fathers' acts were in accord with his own seductive fantasies directed toward his patients, and thus were likely to be fantasy. But he also became more in touch with his fear that his seductive fantasies were having a real seductive effect on his patients and the kind of material they produced. Ultimately he came to doubt the truth of his theories and the truthfulness of his patients. It was his recognition of his seductive impact on their reports, his recognition of his imposition of authority (as Oedipal father, not Oedipal son), that actually led him to abandon the seduction theory. As Freud explains in one of several retrospective accounts: "When, however, I was at last obliged to recognize that these scenes of seduction had never taken place, and that they were only phantasies which my patients had made up or *which I myself had perhaps forced on them,* I was for some time completely at a loss" (italics RBB).[33]

Psychoanalysis (like Freud himself at points) may prefer to blur or downplay the dangers of the analyst imposing his theories and the sense of loss and doubt regarding any future theory that these arouse. Such blurring is facilitated by positing a calm and immediate transition from seduction to Oedipus.

---

[32] R.B. Blass, 'Did Dora have an Oedipus complex – A re-examination of the theoretical context of Freud's "Fragment of an Analysis"', in: *The Psychoanalytic Study of the Child* 47 (1992), pp. 159-187; R.B. Blass & B. Simon, 'Freud on his own mistake(s): The role of seduction in the etiology of neurosis', in: S. Smith & H. Morris (Eds.), *Telling Facts: History and Narration in Psychoanalysis.* Baltimore: Johns Hopkins Press, 1992, pp. 160-183; R.B. Blass & B. Simon, 'The Value of the historical perspective to contemporary psychoanalysis: Freud's "seduction hypothesis"', in: *The International Journal of Psychoanalysis* 75 (1994), pp. 677-693.

[33] Freud, 'Fragment', p. 34.

The second problem that is blurred or perhaps completely lost by positing such a transition allows for is the *problem of sexuality*. Freud put forth many different and at times opposing views on sexuality. The dominant psychoanalytic view regards sexuality as object-related, as the physical origin and expression of love and other forms of personal relatedness. Famously in his '"Wild" Psycho-Analysis' Freud complains (already in 1910) of the misinterpretations and misuses of his ideas on sexuality and specifically of the misunderstanding that by "sexual life" he refers to something somatic, to nothing more than "the need for coitus or analogous acts producing orgasm and emission of the sexual substances".[34] He writes:

> "In psycho-analysis the concept of what is sexual comprises far more; it goes lower and also higher than its popular sense. This extension is justified genetically; we reckon as belonging to 'sexual life' all the activities of the tender feelings which have primitive sexual impulses as their source, even when those impulses have become inhibited in regard to their original sexual aim or have exchanged this aim for another which is no longer sexual. For this reason we prefer to speak of *psychosexuality*, thus laying stress on the point that the mental factor in sexual life should not be overlooked or underestimated. We use the word 'sexuality' in the same comprehensive sense as that in which the German language uses the word *lieben* ['to love']. (…) unsatisfied sexual trends (…) can often find only very inadequate outlet in coitus or other sexual acts.
> Anyone not sharing this view of psychosexuality has no right to adduce psycho-analytic theses dealing with the aetiological importance of sexuality."[35]

But for many years Freud struggled with another view of sexuality, one which is almost completely detached from object relatedness. This view is most directly expressed in his *Three Essays*, published at the same time as the publication of Dora. There Freud draws the following conclusion:

> "(…) we have been in the habit of regarding the connection between the sexual instinct and the sexual object as more intimate than it in fact is. Experience of the cases that are considered abnormal has shown us that in them the sexual instinct and the sexual object are merely soldered together – a fact which we have been in danger of overlooking in consequence

---

[34] S. Freud, '"Wild" Psycho-Analysis' (1910), *SE* 11, pp. 219-228, p. 222.
[35] Ibid., pp. 222-223.

of the uniformity of the normal picture, where the object appears to form part and parcel of the instinct. We are thus warned to loosen the bond that exists in our thoughts between instinct and object. It seems probable that the sexual instinct is in the first instance independent of its object; nor is its origin likely to be due to its object's attractions."[36]

From this perspective, we come into the world rather with diverse and polymorphously perverse desires, a fairly wild assortment of biologically based tendencies. Conflict occurs between this impersonal heritage and our personal and cultural selves. In his summary at the end of the *Three Essays* Freud writes:

> "In view of what was now seen to be the wide dissemination of tendencies to perversion we were driven to the conclusion that a disposition to perversions is an original and universal disposition of the human sexual instinct and that normal sexual behaviour is developed out of it as a result of organic changes and psychical inhibitions occurring in the course of maturation (…). Among the forces restricting the direction taken by the sexual instinct we laid emphasis upon shame, disgust, pity and the structures of morality and authority erected by society."[37]

Accordingly, the concern with the object is not central, but defensive. An interesting example of this may be seen in one of Freud's letter to Jung in 1907. In this letter, relying on his claim that the "sexual instinct is originally autoerotic" and only later is directed towards objects, he suggests that the hysteric's reports of love and even seduction at an early age may come to conceal the autoerotic trend of the instinct. Freud writes that "hysteria (…) takes as an object anything that bears the remotest relation to a normal object".[38]

In the Dora case Freud is concerned with the role of objects, but also gives considerable room to his non-object-related view of sexuality. For example, the explanation in terms of masturbation has to do with the sexual tendency per se. There is a desire for masturbatory gratification and when that can't find expression then the pathological manifestations ensue. Indeed, this has implications for object relations (e.g., the rejections of the advances of a suitor), but these are not regarded by Freud to be the primary source of the problem.

---

[36] S. Freud, *Three Essays on the Theory of Sexuality* (1905), *SE 7*, pp. 125-243, pp. 147-148.
[37] Ibid., p. 231.
[38] S. Freud, 'Letter from Sigmund Freud to C. G. Jung, Undated', *The Freud/Jung Letters: The Correspondence Between Sigmund Freud and C. G. Jung*, W. McGuire (ed.). Princeton: Princeton University Press, 1974. 38-40, p. 39.

By positing that Dora was an Oedipal case, Freud's complex struggle with his other view of sexuality disappears. Psychoanalysis is spared reflection on the idea of sexuality as something non-object-related and it is spared dealing with the contradiction of this idea with that of sexuality as object-related, which is exemplified by Freud's Oedipal model.

The third and final problem that gets overlooked when Dora is regarded as an Oedipal case is that *in order to shift to the Oedipal model Freud introduces and relies on a theory regarding man's ethical nature*. This is not a theory about what tends to make people *feel* guilty, but rather about how people are actually guilty. I am speaking here of Freud's introduction in *Totem and Taboo* (1913) of the notion of the murder of the primal father at the hand of the rebellious sons and how their sense of guilt for this act is transmitted to all future generations. This notion is essential for Freud's explanation of the universality of the inner Oedipal conflict. In the seduction theories (so called) pathology was thought to emerge from a clash between the person and the traumatic forces of the external world. In the theories of fixation that Freud speaks of in the *Three Essays* and in the Dora case, there is a clash between the desire for infantile sexual gratification (which could not truly be given up because of some kind of external stimulation) and the demands of mature life. But how could there be a clash, a conflict that is inherent to man? For this Freud places an object-related conflicted event at the grounds of human nature. The conflicted love towards the father and the guilt over the destructive attempt to resolve it is ingrained in our DNA, so to speak. This move is problematic because of the questionable historical and genetic theories that are involved here – the legacy of *Totem and Taboo* is one that the analytic community is happy to forget or pervert.[39] But it is also problematic because of the implicit shift to an ethical perspective that this move entails. Psychoanalysis usually prefers to see itself as a purely psychological theory. To be well one must avoid overstimulation that would overwhelm or fixate the psychic mechanism. But with the addition of the idea that the mind is shaped by guilt-arousing conflictual relationships that *actually* occurred in prehistory to be well one must also acknowledge guilt, wrong-doing at least in terms of one's wishes, and find a way to deal with it. Here too, by postulating an early and easy transition to his Oedipal model psychoanalysis is spared contending with these problematic issues.

---

[39] R.B. Blass, 'The role of tradition in concealing and grounding truth: Two opposing Freudian legacies on truth and tradition', in: *American Imago* 63 (2006), pp. 331-353.

Conclusion

Having described how misreading Dora as one of Freud's Oedipal cases makes life easier, spares psychoanalysis encounter with some very thorny issues that go to the very heart of psychoanalytic thinking and practice, I would like to conclude by affirming (what may be obvious) that this is not a good thing. As psychoanalysis has taught us, it is by encountering the complexity of reality, the difficulties and conflicts inherent to it, that our thinking and our lives are enriched. In this instance a fuller appreciation of the meaning and value of the Oedipus complex is made possible by recognizing, not overlooking, the difficult steps involved in its adoption. The Dora case provides us an opening to view Freud in the midst of his struggle.

Sexuality and Knowledge in Dora's Case

Beatriz Santos

In the afterword to 'Fragments of an Analysis of a Case of Hysteria', Freud formulates a theoretical orientation that is still reiterated by psychoanalysts today: "I can only repeat over and over again – for I never find it otherwise – that sexuality is the key to the problem of the psychoneuroses and of the neuroses in general. No one who disdains the key will ever be able to unlock the door".[1] The understanding of the afflictions studied by Freud in the early stages of psychoanalysis, and particularly the understanding of hysteria, is directly tied to an understanding of sexuality. Whoever does not take into account the way in which the sexual and psychic lives are tied cannot pretend to practice psychoanalysis.

But which sexuality is Freud referring to when writing this text, commonly called by its protagonist's name, Dora? What does Freud know about sexuality when he writes the story of this analysis? What can we say of these theories that, in spite of preceding the publication of the *Three Essays on the Theory of Sexuality*, seem to already put forth certain key concepts of the 1905 text? These questions on the beginnings of the construction of the notion of *sexuality* will guide the discussions presented in this article. They will also direct our reflection on two other issues at work in Dora's treatment: that of the existence of a *hysterical disposition*, and that of the *fragments* of an analysis.

Dream and hysteria

When Freud meets Dora, in October of 1900, he has already published *The Interpretation of Dreams* (1900). At this moment he wishes to write about a case that could serve as an example of the practical application of the theories he presented there. In the foreword to 'Fragment of an Analysis of a Case of Hysteria', he states his intention to name the article 'Dream and Hysteria', since it is a treatment in which the importance of the interpretation of dreams is easily demonstrated. It is the interpretation of the two dreams told by Dora that allows Freud to elucidate the symptoms and to fill in Dora's amnesias: it confirms in Freud's eyes the importance of dreams as an access to unconscious content, unattainable otherwise.

---

[1] S. Freud, 'Fragment of an Analysis of a Case of Hysteria' (1905 [1901]), *SE* 7, p. 115.

Indeed, in a letter sent to Fliess on January 25th 1901, Freud describes his perception of Dora's case as follows:

> "I finished "Dream and Hysteria" yesterday, and today I already miss a narcotic. It is a fragment of an analysis of a case of hysteria in which the explanations are grouped around two dreams; so it is really a continuation of the dream book. In addition, it contains resolutions of hysterical symptoms and glimpses of the sexual-organic foundation of the whole. It is the subtlest thing I have written so far and *will put people off even more than usual*. Still, one does one's duty and does not write for the day alone."[2]

Dora's analysis is then a work in which dreams take a capital place, and it is also a work which will put off Freud's readers. Let us take a brief closer look at these two points.

Freud reaffirms in the conclusion to his text that one of his goals was to show that the art of dream interpretation "can be turned to account for the discovery of the hidden and repressed parts of mental life".[3] Dora's analysis rests on two dreams. The first is a recurring dream in which "a house is on fire". Dora's father is standing in front of her bed and wakes her up, and Dora gets dressed quickly. Her mother still wants to save her jewelry box, so the father tells her he doesn't want his two children, as well as himself, to burn because of this object. They go down and exit the house. Dora wakes up. For Freud, the hidden content that the dream made explicit was Dora's masturbatory activity when she was a child.

In the second dream, Dora is walking in a foreign city. When she comes back home, she finds a letter from her mother telling her that, since Dora left the house unbeknownst to her parents, she (the mother) hadn't wanted to write to tell Dora that her father was ill. But if she wants, she can come back home now to visit him. Dora asks where the train station is and gets "five minutes" as an answer. In front of a thick forest that she enters, there is a young man who tells her: "Still two and a half hours". He wants to accompany her, Dora says no. When she gets home, the maidservant tells her: "Your mother and the others are already at the cemetery".[4]

---

[2] S. Freud, 'Letter from Freud to Fliess, January 25, 1901', in: *The Complete Letters of Sigmund Freud to Wilhelm Fliess* 1887–1904, J.M. Masson (Ed.). Cambridge, MA: The Belknap Press of Harvard University Press, 1985, pp. 432-433 (emphasis added).
[3] Freud, 'Fragment', p. 114.
[4] Ibid., p. 94.

Regarding this second dream, Freud makes three interpretations: he sees in it the confirmation of one of Dora's states of mind (namely, the "maternal longing for a child"[5]); the fulfillment of a gap in her memory (the existence of a maidservant upon whom Mr K. would have made sexual advances); and an explanation for the formation of the symptom of her dragging one leg. The description of the path towards each of these discoveries constitutes a great part of the record of this analysis. And Freud also describes Dora's reaction to these interpretations: "At the end of the second session, when I expressed my satisfaction at the result, Dora replied in a depreciatory tone: 'Why, has anything so very remarkable come out?'".[6] Throughout her brief analysis, Dora was always in disagreement with Freud's interpretations. But that did not change the orientation Freud gave to the treatment, which surprises certain commentators of the Freudian text – particularly those who confront it with other references outside of psychoanalytical theory.[7]

Let us now turn to the repelling aspect that Freud attributes to this case story ("It is the subtlest thing I have written so far and *will put people off even more than usual*"). When Freud talks of *putting* people off, he is referring to the fact that "sexual questions will be discussed with all possible frankness, the organs and functions of sexual life will be called by their proper names" in his text.[8] And he continues with a warning: "the pure-minded reader can convince himself from my description that I have not hesitated to converse upon such subjects in such language even with a young woman".[9] Freud knows that the description of a treatment should not omit the words heard during the sessions, just as he knows that those words can shock unaware readers by their connection to sexual life. That is why he uses the foreword to present his point of view on the stakes of writing such a case. This is about respecting his duty towards science, and not only his duty towards his patients, which means to publish what he believes he knows of the causes and structure of hysteria, for the benefit of other patients who suffer of the same illness. The text's foreword is thus the place to, in his words, justify from various standpoints the steps taken, and to partly diminish the expectations to which it will give rise.[10]

---

[5] Ibid., p. 104.
[6] Ibid.
[7] See e.g. C. Berheimer & C. Kahane (Eds.), *In Dora's Case. Freud, Hysteria, Feminism*. New York: Columbia University Press, 1990. For a psychoanalytical approach to this question, see the work of Patrick Mahony, *Freud's Dora. A Psychoanalytic, Historical and Textual Study*. New Haven: Yale University Press, 1996.
[8] Freud, 'Fragment', p. 9.
[9] Ibid.
[10] Ibid., p. 7.

This certainty regarding the legitimacy of his practice, in other words, the fact that Freud knows for a fact that talking about sexuality to a patient is not a way to satiate sexual desires, doesn't keep him from worrying about the "repulsive" character of his text. And that mention to the frightened reaction of some of his readers must be understood in two ways. It is first of all a reaction related to the norms organizing Viennese society in Freud's time. Of course, Freud is aware of the fact that a psychoanalyst addressing matters related to sexuality in a direct manner with an eighteen-year-old woman might shock early-twentieth-century readers. But that someone should assume that talking about sex in analysis is a way of satisfying sexual desires that would stand as "the mark of a singular and perverse prurience". This means it is the indication of something that is not solved by more modesty in the text, since it is another type of problem entirely.

Which brings us to the other side of the repulsed reaction Freud anticipates. This reaction is also a response coherent with the neurosis of his readers. As he points out, reading the description of a treatment largely based on the work of interpreting dreams demands of the reader a familiarity with the procedure. Should one not know how psychoanalysis works, reading about it – and specially reading a clinical example of it – would not convince, but rather *disconcert* the reader. It is the normal neurotic reaction to that which is not yet familiar: fear or embarrassment. Dora's analysis – as all analyses published by Freud – lead the reader to "assume the existence of many new things."[11] And "What is new has always aroused bewilderment and resistance."[12]

More precisely, Freud's consideration of the readers' reactions when faced with the sexual aspects of Dora's case may well be seen as a metapsychological problem. It describes a *transposition* effect happening between the analytical work and its text: namely, the fact that the exposition of a psychoanalytical topic can be an integral part of the very thing it is describing. This means that what Freud says about the unconscious is as much an exposition *on* the unconscious as it is an exposition *of* the unconscious. Pierre Fédida describes this as the "transformability criterion", *critère de transformabilité* proper to psychoanalytical theory – "the operation of transformation authorized by the idea of theory: from sexual theory [*Sexualtheorie*] to the theory of sexuality, or from dream theory [*Traumtheorie*] to the dream as theory".[13]

---

[11] Ibid., p. 10.
[12] Ibid.
[13] P. Fédida, 'Technique psychanalytique et métapsychologie', in: *Métapsychologie et Philosophie*. Paris: Belles Lettres, 1985, p. 46 (our translation).

Theories of sexuality before 1905

In a text on Charcot's work and the history of psychiatry in the modern age, Mark S. Micale stressed that "the period 1870 and 1910 witnessed an unprecedented burst of creative psychological theorizing in Europe and the United States. This was the founding generation of modern psychology, psychiatry, and psychotherapy during which the sciences of the mind largely assumed the theoretical and professional forms in which we know them today".[14] Freud's sexual theories are an important part of this creative expansion of clinical sciences. And similarly to what Micale describes in the history of psychiatry, inside the Freudian body of work certain ideas presented during that founding period (before 1910) still maintain their innovative character.

One of these first ideas is that of infantile sexuality. In the original text of the *Traumdeutung* Freud refers to the happiness of childhood, which "is still innocent of sexual desire".[15] This reference seems to point to an ignorance of the work of sexual drives in children. That could be confirmed when, a bit further, Freud describes childhood dreams as devoid of interest, as they are mere "wish fulfillments". Does this mean that infantile sexuality (in the sense of perverse activities of the child) is still unknown to Freud? We do not think so. More probably, this sentence in *The Interpretation of Dreams* is an aberration in the text, an affirmation that is not representative of what Freud knows about infantile sexuality at that moment. Indeed, we notice that already from 1896 Freud deals with infantile fantasies of his patients. And throughout the year 1897, the letters to Fliess put forth outlines of concepts that will be part of his text on infantile sexuality, as well as of his sexual theory in general.

We see for instance that in a letter to Fliess dating from November 14 1897,[16] Freud describes his latest discoveries on how the libido operates. Written some years before the *Three Essays*, this text reads as a first draft of the 1905 text, presenting some of its central notions. It indicates aspects of a theory of sexuality that is not yet accomplished, but whose contours we can already guess.

---

[14] M. S. Micale, 'Jean-Martin Charcot and *les névroses traumatiques*: From Medicine to Culture in French Trauma Theory of the Late Nineteen Century', in: M. S. Micale & P. Lerner (Eds.), *Traumatic Pasts: History, Psychiatry, and Trauma in the Modern Age*. Cambridge: Cambridge University Press, 2001, p. 116.
[15] S. Freud, *The Interpretation of Dreams* (1900), SE 4, p. 129.
[16] S. Freud, 'Letter from Freud to Fliess, November 14, 1897', in: *The Complete Letters of Sigmund Freud to Wilhelm Fliess*, pp. 278-282.

First, Freud presents the normal trajectory of the repression of the libido in terms of a consequence of the abandonment of non-genital sexual zones. Throughout their development, the anal and bucco-pharyngian regions lose their place as sites of release for the benefit of an investment in genital zones. The normal development – or, in Freud's words, "the evolving progress" – of the child is understood as this investment in genital organs (at the cost of investment in the mouth and/or anus). This means that the existence of erogenous zones, as well as the variability of their importance throughout a life, is already known in 1897:

> "in infancy the release of sexuality is not yet so much *localized* as it is later, so that the zones which are later abandoned (and perhaps the whole surface of the body as well) also instigate something that is analogous to the later release of sexuality."[17]

The zones that orient one's sexual life are not the same throughout their existence. And, at birth, this very idea of *orientation* has no meaning, since the entire surface of the body is able to be sexually invested. This is what Freud in the *Three Essays on the Theory of Sexuality* will later call the child's polymorphously perverse predisposition. Ultimately, this 1897 letter already contains a reflection on the particular temporality at work in the creation of the symptom, especially the hysterical symptom – namely, the fact that an action taking place in childhood later receives a markedly stronger sexual discharge by a deferred effect of memory.[18]

These three topics (the existence of erogenous zones, the polymorphous predisposition, and the deferred, *après-coup* effect of memory) are also present in Dora's analysis. They represent pieces of the sexual theory on which Freud is counting to simultaneously understand and explain the work done with Dora. More precisely, the importance of these three notions for Dora's analysis reveals the shaping of a sexual theory that will only be available to Freud's readers in 1905. Which means that, despite having already conceived of several notions that will be part of the *Three Essays on the Theory of Sexuality*, he must present Dora's case to readers that don't know this theory yet.

---

[17] Ibid. (emphasis added).
[18] "If a child's genitals have been irritated by someone, years afterward the memory of this will produce by deferred action a release of sexuality far stronger than at the time, because the decisive apparatus and the quota of secretion have increased in the meantime." Ibid., p. 206.

What Freud knows about sexuality is still *fragmentary* when he writes Dora's case. This is why Freud feels obliged, as early as in the Foreword, to insist on the limited scope of his telling.

> "any one who has hitherto been unwilling to believe that a psychosexual aetiology holds good generally and without exception for hysteria is scarcely likely to be convinced of the fact by taking stock of a single case history. He would do better to suspend his judgement until *his own work* has earned him the right to a conviction."[19]

Whoever reads the text won't be convinced by Freud's arguments in favor of a psychosexual cause for hysteria. This is true because, as Lacan will say much later, "*il ne faut pas convaincre – le propre de la psychanalyse, c'est de ne pas vaincre, con ou pas*".[20] In other words, since psychoanalysis is not a scientific investigation but an analytical intervention that doesn't aim to prove anything in itself, the question of its effectiveness may present itself differently than in other fields. Freud cannot produce a demonstration, in the logical sense, of the causal relation between the events that took place in Dora's life and her symptoms. But he does not want to either: the conviction must come from the reader's *own work*.

To this indication of the limits of the text 'Fragment of an Analysis of a Case of Hysteria' – comparable to the limits of any psychoanalytical text – is added the yet fragmentary aspect of the sexual theory in 1900. In the cases presented after 1905, Freud makes direct reference to the explanations given in the *Three Essays on the Theory of Sexuality*. In the 'Analysis of a Phobia in a Five-Year-Old Boy' from 1908, when he describes for the first time the fact that little Hans considers his sister has a small penis that will grow, Freud refers us to the section "The sexual researches of childhood" in the *Three Essays*. And the analysis of the meaning given to feces by the Wolf Man – namely, feces as a gift from the child, or "a portion of his own body which he is ready to part with, but only for the sake of some one he loves" – mentions the text on the activity of the anal zone in children.[21] But Dora's case cannot mention a theory of sexuality because that is not yet completed. Dora's analysis rests on two pillars: the analysis of her dreams and the discovery of psychosexual causes

---

[19] Freud, 'Fragment', p. 13 (emphasis added).
[20] J. Lacan, *Encore. Séminaire XX*, texte établi par J.A. Miller, Paris: Seuil, 1993, p. 50. Lacan's pun (convaincre – convince; con-vaincre – cunt-vanquish) is lost in translation: "one mustn't convince – psychoanalysis' own is to not vanquish, cunt or not."
[21] S. Freud, 'From the History of an Infantile Neurosis' (1918), *SE 17*, p. 80.

of her hysteria. A theory of dreams already exists. But the absence of a sexual theory makes the theorization of Dora's treatment *fragmentary*: it remains waiting for a systematization of the concepts on sexuality.

Organic conditions for hysteria, heredity and the notion of disposition

This idea of a fragmentary theory of sexuality raises the following question: could Freud have treated Dora differently if his notional apparatus had been more developed? It is a matter that has followed the readings of Dora's case for a long time, for at least two reasons. The first is intrinsic to psychoanalytical theory, and comes from the fact that Freud himself presents Dora as a failed analysis. In his words, this means that aspects of the case "prevented results being brought about such as are attainable in other instances, where the improvement will be admitted by the patient and his relatives and will approximate more or less closely to a complete recovery".[22]

The second reason is cultural and concerns the non-psychoanalytical readings of this case. Freud's confession, at the end of his record, that he "failed to discover in time and to inform the patient that her homosexual (gynaecophilic) love for Frau K. was the strongest unconscious current in her mental life"[23] is an example of the themes that have nourished discussions on the Freudian difficulty in listening to his female patients in a way not oriented by a masculine model of sexuality.

Yet, another redefinition of Dora's treatment is not our goal. To imagine new possible readings of the elements presented by Freud is an interesting exercise, but it remains an exercise. It does not in the least change the fact that it was Dora who lay on the couch, and that she told Freud what she did, and that Freud made his interpretations like he made them. What interests us, on the contrary, is to seize the way Freud himself indicates possible theoretical paths from his observations, and how certain paths are chosen while others will later be abandoned. At the outskirts of the themes that progressively become central as psychoanalytical theory advances, each Freudian text opens more leads than it follows. In Dora's analysis, the discussion on organic conditions for hysteria is one of those leads.

In the presentation of Dora's case, Freud declares his intention to question both the somatic evidences of Dora's hysterical trouble and the relational aspect her symptoms may have. He wishes to analyze what he calls *the nature of psychoanalytical facts*:

---

[22] Freud, 'Fragment', p. 114.
[23] Ibid., p. 119.

> "It follows from the nature of the facts which form the material of psycho-analysis that we are obliged to pay as much attention in our case histories to the purely human and social circumstances of our patients as to the somatic data and the symptoms of the disorder."[24]

Dora's case is indeed an opportunity for Freud to return to certain hypotheses concerning the relation between organic conditions and familial stakes at play in hysteria. His first descriptions of Dora, before beginning the treatment, show the importance he attributes to the hereditary aspect of her illness. Freud first knew Dora's father, who came to see him four years before Dora's analysis. On that occasion, Freud had recommended an "energetic anti-syphilitic treatment" that had cured him of his illness.[25] He had also met one of Dora's aunts (who suffered from "a severe form of psychoneurosis, without the characteristic symptoms of a hysteria"[26]), and one of her uncles (a "hypochondriacal bachelor"[27]).

These references to Dora's extended family put forth the question of the role played by heredity, already introduced in the 1896 article 'Heredity and the Aetiology of the Neuroses'.[28] For Freud, some of Dora's characteristics would allow one to see her as part of her family. Those are her intellectual gifts and maturity, and her *predisposition to illness* – which does not mean that hysteria is hereditary. Freud insists, in a long note added to this paragraph on predisposition, that he does not think that "heredity is the only etiology of hysteria". He specifies however that he does not adopt the position that heredity is the only etiological factor in hysteria, even though he does not wish "to give an impression of underestimating the importance of heredity in the etiology of hysteria or of asserting that it can be dispensed with".[29]

Such a reference to heredity brings to light an interesting indication of how the pathogenesis of hysteria is theorized when Freud analyses Dora. How does one become hysteric in 1900? In a recent rereading of Dora's case, Philippe Van Haute and Thomas Geyskens come back to what they describe as the

---

[24] Freud, 'Fragment', p. 17.
[25] Ibid., p. 18.
[26] Ibid.
[27] Ibid.
[28] "As regards nervous heredity, I am far from being able to estimate correctly its influence in the aetiology of the psycho-neuroses. I admit that its presence is indispensable for severe cases; I doubt if it is necessary for slight ones; but I am convinced that nervous heredity by itself is unable to produce psychoneuroses if their specific aetiology, precocious sexual excitation, is missing. I even believe that the decision as to which of the neuroses, hysteria or obsessions, will develop in a given case, is not decided by heredity but a special characteristic of the sexual event in earliest childhood." S. Freud, 'Heredity and the Aetiology of the Neuroses' (1896), *SE 3*, p. 155.
[29] Ibid., p. 19.

specific etiology of hysteria.[30] Their work analyses the importance of psychical reality and of fantasy productions in Dora's treatment, and confront it with the oedipal explanation traditionally given for it. More precisely, Van Haute and Geyskens invite us to come back to Freud's first steps in order to resize the importance of the Oedipus in Dora's hysteria. According to them, between 1895 and 1905 Freud developed a theory on hysteria that is not centered around oedipal stakes. One of the arguments demonstrating this is the absence of references to the Oedipus complex in the text of the 'Fragment'.[31] According to Van Haute and Geyskens, "between 1987 and 1905, Freud's theory of neurosis is characterized by a number of displacements in the relations between accidental and constitutional factors in the *specific* etiology of hysteria".[32] This means that, in this first formulating moment of the theory of hysteria (and of psychoanalytical theory in general), Freud is dealing with the problem of the hysterical disposition. Does one become hysterical because of a traumatic (and accidental) experience, or is one predisposed to hysteria (by one's constitution)? For Van Haute and Geyskens, when Freud meets Dora he decides in favor of the predisposition hypothesis, and sees hysteria as an incurable tendency, an essential part of human existence.[33]

Van Haute and Geyskens also stress that it is not the oedipal problem that orients Dora's hysteria, but rather her bisexuality. Her symptoms tie in with the originally bisexual predisposition, that is, the possibility to have men as well as women as love objects before the setting of the oedipal organization. Freud insists on the (oedipal) love of Dora for Mr K. (for instance when he states that "her illness was therefore a demonstration of her love for K., just as his wife's was a demonstration of her *dislike*"[34]). This determination keeps him from listening to what Dora says of her love for Mrs K., the appreciation she had for her tastes, as well as her attraction to her "adorable white body".[35]

The repeated attempts to affirm Dora's oedipal heterosexuality are in part oriented by the cultural context in which this analysis happened. But it is not only Freud's inability to consider that Dora is a lesbian that has him reading her

---

[30] Ph. Van Haute & T. Geyskens, *A Non-OedipalPpsychoanalysis? A Clinical Anthropology of Hysteria in the Works of Freud and Lacan*, Leuven: Leuven University Press, 2012.

[31] There is indeed a single reference to the fable of Oedipus in all the text of Dora's case: "I have shown at length elsewhere [in the *Interpretation of Dreams*] at what an early age sexual attraction makes itself felt between parents and children, and I have explained that the legend of Oedipus is probably to be regarded as a poetical rendering of what is typical in these relations". Freud, 'Fragment', p. 55.

[32] Van Haute & Geyskens, *A Non-oedipal Psychoanalysis?*, p. 27.

[33] Ibid.

[34] Freud, 'Fragment', p. 39.

[35] Ibid., p. 60.

desires under an Oedipus-centered perspective. For Van Haute and Geyskens, what is at work is Freud's intention to "protect him from the *structural dissolution of gender identities* that result from a general disposition towards bisexuality".[36] In other words, Freud wishes to be able to say that Dora has an identifiable desire (for a man) with a known source (the love for her father). But this certitude is incompatible with the bisexual hypothesis.

Fragments of a conclusion

There are three reasons to consider Dora's case as *fragments* of an analysis, according to Freud. The first stems from the fact that the case is based on a theory of sexuality which, on the one hand, is not yet written by Freud (since the *Three Essays* will only be published five years later) and which, on the other, is marked by the operation of transformation characteristic of the fabrication of concepts pertaining to sexuality, as we argued earlier. In other words, those are indeed fragments of the analysis because the theory of sexuality is not yet completed by Freud in 1900 – but also because Freud's project to establish univocal relations between causes and effects in sexuality will not come to fruition. It will always need to be followed by the reader's "own work", as Freud puts it. This is why we are told that a single patient story cannot address all the questions raised by an analysis, because only the work of the treatment can make explicit the importance of psychosexual causes in the formation of symptoms.[37]

The second reason for which Freud mentions the idea of fragments is the fact that Dora's analysis is one that did not reach its end:

> "the treatment was not carried through to its appointed end, but was broken off at the patient's own wish when it had reached a certain point. At that time some of the problems of the case had not even been attacked and others had only been imperfectly elucidated; whereas, if the work had been continued, we should no doubt have obtained the fullest possible enlightenment upon every particular of the case. In the following pages, therefore, I can present only a fragment of an analysis."[38]

The story or *récit* of this treatment differs from other studies which allow Freud to thoroughly describe his interpretation work – such as the Wolf Man case, where he is able to establish a detailed description of the dream followed by a "comprehensive account of the relations between the manifest content of

---

[36] Van Haute & Geyskens, *A Non-Oedipal Psychoanalysis?*, p. 58 (emphasis added).
[37] Freud, 'Fragment', p. 12.
[38] Ibid., p. 11.

the dream and the latent dream-thoughts".[39] But Dora's precociously interrupted treatment obliges Freud to present a "mutilated" material, which he must then complete in order to analyze, like an archaeologist reconstructing pieces found in a search site.

Lastly, Freud talks about *fragments* to describe his new way of presenting his interpretations. In the earliest treatments, the analytical work consisted of starting from the symptoms and trying to 'solve' them one after another. This is what we see in the *Studies on Hysteria*. But Dora's analysis comes after a 'revolution' of the technique, as described by Freud: the abandonment of hypnosis in favor of the technique of free association: "I now let the patient himself choose the subject of the day's work, and in that way I start out from whatever surface his unconscious happens to be presenting to his notice at the moment".[40]

The consequence of this new technique is a "disorder" of the material worked on by Freud: the material "emerges piecemeal, woven into various contexts, and distributed over widely separated periods of time". In other words, it is a fragmented material. Which demands a different work on the analyst's part, who must now "complete that which is incomplete". The work required is no longer to bring to light the memory of the event causing the hysteric symptom, as it was the case in the first treatments, but rather to provide *constructions* that turn these fragments into understandable material to the patient – and to the reader.

But this description of the analysis in terms of a work on fragments must not be radically opposed to the idea of a totality. When Freud describes the fragments of an analysis, he is also describing how each one of the pieces is a unity in itself, how there is value in each one of them. If it is true that each fragment is clarified when Freud establish a comprehensive account, we must also consider that such a view in itself is also fragmentary in relation to psychoanalysis. More precisely, the fragment of an analysis – the memory of a dream, the slip produced in a session – is a unity we examine for itself. And such a unity takes its full meaning in relation to another unity: that of the finished analysis. Yet, every finished analysis can be seen as the fragment of an analyst and an analysand's experience. Even when it is finished, the analysis is not a totality – which is why Pierre Fédida spoke of the *trans-finite* dimension of the cure, that is of an end that is also the origin of a work: "an analytical treatment can and must receive an end (a termination) when it has established in the analyst *the conditions for an unending analytical activity* – transfinite, so

---

[39] Freud, 'From the History of an Infantile Neurosis', p. 41.
[40] Freud, 'Fragment', p. 11.

to speak".[41] Such an activity includes the ability to revise and modify certitudes about all that constitutes an analysis. It finds its echo in the thought processes that a case story as rich as Dora's invites us to accomplish, over a hundred years after her last session.

---

[41] P. Fédida, *Le site de l'étranger*, Paris: PUF, 1995, p. 301.

Trauma and Disgust:
Dora between Freud and Laplanche

Philippe Van Haute

'Fragment of an Analysis of a Case of Hysteria' ('The Dora case') is structured around two dreams that played a crucial role in the analysis of Dora who suffered from a *petite hystérie*.[1] In the last years of the 19th century, Freud studied dreams extensively and he published his *Interpretation of Dreams* in the last months of 1899.[2] Freud became interested in the processes governing the formation of dreams because he was convinced, as he states in the beginning of the 'Fragment', that "the dream is one of the roads along which consciousness can be reached by the psychic material which, on account of the opposition aroused by its content, has been cut off from consciousness and repressed, and has thus been pathogenic".[3] The mechanisms employed in our dreams to evade repression – displacement, condensation etcetera – are analogous to those that govern symptom formation. Freud is interested in dreams because they help him understand neurotic symptom formation.[4] But dreams also have a clinical significance within the therapy: "these dreams seemed to call for insertion in the long thread of connections which spun itself out between a symptom of a disease and a pathogenic idea".[5] The dreams told to him by patients were indeed crucial to understanding the unconscious ideas at the basis of neurotic pathology. 'Fragment of an Analysis of a Case of Hysteria' sets out to illustrate precisely this clinical significance of dreams.[6]

The study of dreams allowed Freud to articulate the basic psychological mechanisms determining the symptomatology of neurosis, in particular of hysteria. But Freud never considered psychoanalysis to be an exclusively psychological theory. In his famous letter from September 17, 1897 in which he announces that he no longer believes in his 'neurotica' – and hence in an exclusively psychological theory of neurosis – he also states that this abandonment once again brings the hereditary and constitutional aspects of neurosis to the

---
[1] S. Freud, 'Fragment of an Analysis of a Case of Hysteria' (1905 [1901]), *SE* 7, p. 23.
[2] S. Freud, The Interpretation of Dreams (1900), *SE 4-5*.
[3] Freud, 'Fragment', p. 15.
[4] Ibid., pp. 10-11.
[5] Ibid., p. 15.
[6] Ibid., p. 15. All of this also explains why Freud originally wanted to call the Dora case 'Dreams and hysteria' (Ibid., p. 10).

fore.⁷ It is clear that Freud first counted on Fliess to articulate the biological foundations of neurosis. But Fliess did not provide him with such a theory. On the contrary, it took Freud's own *Three Essays on the Theory of Sexuality*, published in the same year as the 'Fragment', to elaborate this theory. The *Three Essays* articulate a hysterical constitution or disposition that is at the basis of hysteria proper. Freud stresses that the basic elements of this constitution – infantile (perverse) sexuality, bisexuality etc. – characterize human sexuality as such. Nobody really escapes from hysteria.⁸

How then does the 'Fragment of an Analysis of a Case of Hysteria' fits into this double reference to psychology and biology? Freud writes: "[the history of the treatment of a hysterical girl] will at the same time give me a first opportunity of publishing at sufficient length to prevent further misunderstanding some of my views upon the psychical processes and upon its organic determinants".⁹ From here it becomes possible to adequately understand the meaning of the reference to the *Studies on Hysteria* – and hence to the trauma theory of neurosis – that we find in the Dora case. Freud explains: "Since then (since the publication of the *Studies*) I have seen an abundance of cases of hysteria, and I have been occupied with each case for a number of days, weeks, or years. In not a single one of them have I failed to discover the psychological determinants which were postulated in the *Studies*, namely, a psychological trauma, a conflict of affects, and an additional factor which I brought forward in later publications – a disturbance in the sphere of sexuality".¹⁰ The 'additional factor' alluded to here is precisely what is explained at great length in the *Three Essays*.¹¹ Hence it makes sense to read the 'Dora case' to show that psychological factors ('trauma') and mechanisms (displacement...) can only be understood against the background of 'organic ('sexual') determinants' characterizing human sexuality as such.¹² This also means that the 'Fragment' allows us to understand the clinical

---

⁷ *The Complete Letters of Sigmund Freud to Wilhelm Fliess* 1887–1904, J.M. Masson (Ed.). Cambridge, MA: The Belknap Press of Harvard University Press 1985, p. 264.
⁸ S. Freud, *Three Essays on the Theory of Sexuality*, SE 7, p. 171.
⁹ Freud, 'Fragment', p. 15.
¹⁰ Ibid., p. 24.
¹¹ S. Freud, 'My Views on the Part played by Sexuality in the Aetiology of the Neuroses' (1906), SE 7, p. 276.
¹² Speaking of the development of his thought after 1897, Freuds writes in 'My views on the Part played by Sexuality in the Aetiology of the Neuroses': "Accidental influences derived from experience having thus receded into the background, the factors of constitution and heredity necessarily took the upper hand once more; but there was this difference between my views and those prevailing in other quarters, that on my theory the 'sexual constitution' took the place of a general neuropathic disposition". Freud, 'My Views', pp. 275-276.

importance of some of the basic insights of *Three Essays*. In what follows I will try to elucidate the intrinsic link between Dora's hysterical constitution and the traumatic rejection of sexuality that characterizes her pathology.

Une petite hystérie

It is interesting to note that Freud choses 'Dora' to illustrate his clinical and theoretical views on hysteria. Hysteria as it was diagnosed in the second half of the 19th century and the beginning of the 20th century is forever linked to the work of Charcot and to the patients whom he made famous (and who made him famous).[13] However, Dora does not resemble Charcot's hysterical patients with their spectacular symptomatology: hysterical fits, delusional experiences and dramatic conversion symptoms. Compared to Charcot's patients, there is not much that is spectacular about Dora's case. Dora does not suffer from convulsions and she only has minor conversion symptoms: a cough that does not go way, periodic aphonia, some migraine attacks, enuresis and depressive feelings.[14] Freud qualifies her pathological condition as a *petite hystérie* so as to distinguish it from Charcot's *grande hystérie*.

In many respects, Freud's approach here anticipates Bleuler's approach to *dementia praecox* a few years later. Bleuler claimed that in order to understand *dementia praecox*, or schizophrenia as he called it, we don't have to look at the spectacular 'positive' symptoms (delusions, et cetera), but rather at the 'negative' symptoms (apathy, anhedonia, et cetera).[15] Freud makes a similar case with regard to hysteria, stating that in order to understand hysteria we should not look at the rare and amazing phenomena (convulsions…), but at the average cases that present the most common, typical symptoms.[16] What characterizes hysteria more than anything else, so he claims, is a 'negative' symptom in a sense close to those elaborated by Bleuler. Hysterical patients are no longer capable of enjoying sexuality. Hysteria is fundamentally characterized by a spontaneous and pre-representational disgustful rejection of sexuality: "I should without question consider a person hysterical in whom an occasion for sexual excitement elicited feelings that were preponderantly or exclusively unpleasurable; and I should do so whether or not the person were capable of producing somatic symptoms".[17] From this perspective, understanding hysteria means first and

---

[13] G. Didi-Huberman, *The Invention of Hysteria*. Cambridge (MA)/London: MIT Press, 2003.
[14] Freud, 'Fragment', p. 24.
[15] E. Bleuler, *Dementia Praecox oder die Gruppe der Schizophrenien*. Leipzig: Deuticke, 1911.
[16] Freud, 'Fragment', p. 139.
[17] Ibid., p. 28.

foremost understanding the spontaneous 'reversal of affect' – from pleasure to disgust – that defines it.[18]

Dora rejects sexuality – she is disgusted by it – because it is associated with the excremental.[19] In *Three Essays on the Theory of Sexuality* Freud argues that one of the main tasks with which every human being is confronted consists in overcoming the link between the sexual and the excremental.[20] Freud repeats this view in his text on Dora. He writes that disgust is originally the reaction towards the smell and later the sight of excrement. Furthermore, the genitals can act as a reminder of the excretory functions. This is especially true with regard to the male member because that organ is also used to urinate. Freud continues: "Thus it happens that disgust becomes one of the means of affective expression in the sphere of sexual life. The Early Christian Fathers '*inter urinas et faeces nascimur*' cling to sexual life and cannot be detached from it in spite of every effort of idealization".[21] The possibility of a contamination of the sexual by the excremental is an intrinsic element of human sexuality we all have to deal with: "It is scarcely possible to exaggerate the pathogenic significance of the comprehensive tie uniting the sexual and the excremental, a tie which is at the basis of a very large number of hysterical phobias".[22] But 'possibility' is not 'necessity'. Most people manage to produce the psychic work (idealization) necessary to keep sexuality apart from the excremental function. "A knowledge of the paths", Freud states, "does not render less necessary a knowledge of the forces which travel along them".[23] Hence, understanding the disgust for sexuality that is the 'shibboleth' of hysteria implies understanding the forces that led to the *actual* contamination of the sexual by the excremental.

The role of masturbation

I cannot go into all the details of this extremely complex case. Instead, I will concentrate on Freud's remarks on the origin of Dora's disgust for sexuality. This disgust occurred for the first time when Mr K., a friend of the family's

---

[18] Freud further explains that the disgust Dora feels when Mr K. embraces her in his shop also implies a displacement of sensation: "Instead of the genital sensation which would certainly have been felt by a healthy girl in such circumstances, Dora was overcome by the unpleasurable feeling which is proper to the tract of the mucous membrane at the entrance to the alimentary canal – that is by disgust" (Ibid., p. 29). I will come back to this point later.
[19] Ibid., pp. 31-32; pp. 83-84.
[20] Freud, *Three Essays*, p. 152.
[21] Freud, 'Fragment', p. 31.
[22] Ibid., p. 32 – in note.
[23] Ibid., p. 32.

whom she had long fancied,[24] embraces her and tries to kiss her when he was alone with her in his shop.[25] Freud writes that Dora, who was fourteen at the time, felt at that very moment Mr K.'s erect penis against her body.[26] Freud's supposition is that Dora must have felt an analogous change in her clitoris. But she did not feel any pleasure. Instead, this experience was repulsive for her and caused nothing but disgust. Disgust is identified by Freud as the symptom of repression in the oral zone. Hence, we not only find a reversal of affect, but this reversal goes along with a displacement from the genitals to the oral zone. Freud explains this displacement by stressing that as a child Dora was a frenetic thumb sucker, which he links to Dora's lifelong preference for oral pleasures. The latter is an essential element of Dora's sexual constitution. Orality and the oral zone are important to all of us, but in some it is more predominant then in others.

Shortly after the event in the shop, Dora produces the first of the two dreams that structure this case study. She dreams that her family's house is on fire and within the dream she is woken to her father leaning over her. Her mother doesn't want to leave the house without first saving her jewelry box/jewel case. The father replies, however: "I refuse to let my two children be burnt for the sake of your jewel case".[27] Freud considers this dream a reaction to the traumatic event that occurred some days before,[28] but along with his interpretation of this dream, he also gives some crucial elements on the origin of Dora's disgust. According to Freud, this affective reaction does not have a sufficient grounding in the traumatic event itself. On the contrary, since Dora fancied Mr K., she should, according to Freud, have felt pleasure and excitement rather than disgust. Dora's reaction is in a certain sense inconsistent – she simply rejects what she should actually be longing for, given her long-standing love for Mr K. – and this inconsistency requires further explanation.[29]

Not only does the trauma just discussed conceal the affective reversal that characterizes hysteria, but there are also a number of other symptoms predating this trauma. Consistent with the importance accorded by him to the role of trauma in pathology, Freud writes: *"If therefore the trauma theory is not to be abandoned*, we must go back to her childhood and look about there for any influences or impressions which might have had an effect analogous to that

---

[24] Ibid., p. 37.
[25] Ibid., p. 28.
[26] Ibid., p. 30.
[27] Ibid., p. 64.
[28] Ibid.
[29] S. Freud, *Three Essays on the Theory of Sexuality: The 1905 Edition*, Ph. Van Haute & H. Westerink (Eds.); U. Kistner (Transl.). London: Verso, 2016, p. 38 – in note; p. 46; p. 58 (*SE 7*, 176, 185, 205).

of a trauma" (italics PvH).[30] What then does the dream of the burning house teach Freud about 'influences or impressions which might have had an effect analogous to that of a trauma' and that are at the basis of Dora's rejection of sexuality?

In the dream under discussion here, Dora's father is protecting her from the burning fire. According to Freud, the 'fire' refers not just to the burning house, but also to Dora's love for Mr K.: she is 'on fire and in flames' for him. In the dream Dora's father wakes her up, just as he did when she was a child, to prevent her from wetting her bed. Freud concludes that Dora wants her father to protect her from her desire and love for Mr K. just as he used to protect her when she was a child.[31]

But for our purposes, the main question here, according to Freud, is why Dora started bed-wetting again after her sixth year.[32] Strange as this may sound to modern ears, Freud links bed-wetting of this kind explicitly to masturbation. Children know this very well themselves, Freud explains, and Dora is no exception. Freud recalls that Dora explicitly blamed her father for her disease. She had overheard her parents talk about her father's syphilis[33] and she also heard an old aunt remind her mother that 'he was already ill before their marriage'. The aunt added some remarks that Dora didn't understand, but she related them to 'indecent things' at a later stage. Dora concluded that her father became sick because of his frivolous lifestyle and she assumed that he transferred his disease to her through heredity.[34] When Dora accompanies her mother, then suffering from abdominal pains and a discharge (a catarrh), to a spa in Franzensbad, she once again assumes that her father had caused this problem and that he had passed his sexually transmitted infection to her mother. According to Freud, Dora makes the mistake common among lay persons, of confusing gonorrhea

---

[30] Freud, 'Fragment', p. 27.
[31] Ibid., p. 70. It is clear from this that an oedipal reading of the Dora case is not justified. The infantile love for the father is reactivated to ward off Dora's actual love for Mr K. It is this actual love that is at the center of Dora's problematic, and not a repressed love for the father. (That would by the same token explain the disgust.) The father here replaces Mr K. and not the other way around, as would be the case in an oedipal interpretation. On this point, see also Ph. Van Haute & T. Geyskens, 'Between disposition, Trauma and History. How Oedipal was Dora?, in: J. De Vleminck & E. Dorfman (Eds.), *Sexuality and psychoanalysis. Philosophical criticisms*. Leuven: Leuven University Press, 2010.
[32] Freud, 'Fragment', p. 74. See also Freud, *Three Essays*, p. 190.
[33] Freud, 'Fragment', p. 75. It is worth noting that Freud also mentions the importance of the old thesis of degeneracy in this context. Freud's break with past theories is sometimes less radical than we read in the literature: "I was careful not to tell her that, as I already mentioned, I too was of the opinion that the offspring of luetics were very specially predisposed to severe neuropsychoses" (Ibid.). See also Freud, *Three Essays*, p. 236.
[34] Freud seems at least a partially of the same opinion. See previous note.

and syphilis, contamination and hereditary transmission. Dora's identification with her mother on this occasion makes Freud wonder whether Dora did not contract a sexually transmitted infection herself. He then finds out that she is suffering from a catarrh (leucorrhoea) of which she doesn't remember when it started.[35] Leucorrhea, Freud tells Dora, should essentially be understood as a result of masturbation.

Freud concludes from all of this that Dora's accusations against her father are in fact self-accusations, and that she is "now on the way to finding an answer to her own question of why it was that precisely she has fallen ill – by confessing that she had masturbated, probably in childhood".[36] Dora consciously refutes Freud's explanation, but Freud interprets a highly significant 'symptomatic act' – Dora brought a 'small reticule' to the session and "as she lay on the sofa and talked, she kept playing with it – opening it, putting a finger into it, shutting it again, and so on"[37] – as an unconscious confirmation of his conclusion. Masturbation is the one secret that Dora did not want to disclose to her doctors and about which she did not want to talk with anybody.[38]

The analysis of the first dream allows in Freud's opinion to determine the crucial role masturbation played in Dora's history. But how exactly can this role be determined? Freud reminds us that Dora's bed-wetting which he considers to have been caused by masturbation, lasted until shortly before the appearance of her 'nervous asthma' (dyspnoea) when she was eight years old. Freud continues: "Hysterical symptoms hardly ever appear so long as children are masturbating, but only afterwards, when a period of abstinence has set in; they form a substitute for masturbatory satisfaction…".[39] This means that the symptoms that Dora developed before the first trauma when she was fourteen years old have to be understood as substitutes for masturbation (sexual activity). Understanding Dora's pathology means understanding why she gave up masturbation – and this comes down to the question why sexuality became problematic and ultimately disgusting for her. This is completely in line with Freud's characterization of the core (negative) symptom of hysteria: the disgust for sexual pleasure. The central problem to understanding Dora's pathology thus becomes: why did she give up masturbation? Or better still, what trauma lies at the basis of the abandonment of masturbation?

---

[35] Freud, 'Fragment', pp. 75-76.
[36] Ibid., p. 76.
[37] Ibid.
[38] Ibid., p. 78.
[39] Ibid., p. 79.

The original scene

I already referred to the continuity between Freud's theory in the 'Fragment' and his early texts from the end of the 19th century. In the context discussed here, Freud refers once again to his early work and more particularly to his paper on anxiety neurosis from 1895,[40] in which he linked dyspnoea and palpitations in hysteria to detached fragments of the act of copulation. Indeed, according to Freud, Dora's symptomatic acts and some other signs that he does not specify, allow him to conclude that Dora overheard her parents having sexual intercourse. Dora must have divined the sexual nature of the sounds that came from her parents' room since "the movements expressive of sexual excitement lie within them (children, PvH) ready to hand, as innate pieces of mechanism".[41] And Freud concludes: "The sympathetic excitement which may be supposed to have occurred in Dora on such an occasion may very easily have made the child's sexuality veer round and have replaced her inclination to masturbation by an inclination to anxiety".[42]

But why would this be the case? Freud does not really elaborate this point in 'Fragment of an Analysis of a Case of Hysteria', but maybe the *Three Essays* published in the same year as the 'Fragment', can help us here. In *Three Essays* Freud explained at great length that infantile sexuality is autoerotic, that it is without an object and hence also without fantasy (*'objektlos'*).[43] In 1905 infantile sexuality is, in other words, understood in exclusively physiological terms.[44] This can explain why the sexual excitement that Dora experiences when overhearing her parents cannot be bound to adequate (sexual) representations. As a result, the libidinal tension released at this occasion remains free-floating in Dora's psyche. Free-floating libido, Freud already declared in his 1895 text on anxiety neurosis, is transformed into anxiety. This explains how the primal scene is the traumatic confrontation that turns sexuality into an object of anxiety, rather than a source of pleasure.

---

[40] S. Freud, 'On the Grounds for detaching a Particular Syndrome from Neurasthenia under the Description "Anxiety Neurosis"' (1895), *SE 3*.
[41] Freud. 'Fragment', p. 80.
[42] Ibid., p. 80.
[43] Freud, *Three Essays (1905)*, pp. 42-43 (*SE 7*, pp. 181-183). It is important to refer in this context to the first edition of *Three* Essays recently translated into English by Ulrike Kistner (see footnote 29), since it is only in this edition that Freud radically defends the non-objectal status of infantile sexuality. Without this non-objectal (autoerotic) status, the logic of the *Fragment*-text can not really be understood.
[44] Ph. Van Haute & H. Westerink, 'Introduction: Hysteria, Sexuality and the Deconstruction of Normativity', in: Freud, *Three Essays 1905*, xiii-lxxvi.

In the context that concerns me here, Freud notes that Dora at some later stage reproduced 'the impression she had received' while overhearing her parents' sexual activities as an asthma attack. Dora was missing her tenderly beloved father while he was away on business. According to Freud, Dora's unconscious reasoning on this occasion can easily be reconstructed if we take the event that caused the first appearance of the symptom as our starting point. The first attack came at a moment when she was out of breath after a walk in the mountains.[45] From here, a complex chain of reasoning ensues: her father, suffering from shortness of breath, was forbidden to climb in the mountains so as not to over-exert himself; but did he not over-exert himself with her mother the night that Dora overheard them? And, finally, did she not over-exert herself in turn when masturbating? After all, this activity was also accompanied by shortness of breath. Finally, the dyspnoea returned as an intensified symptom expressing her identification with her father.[46]

But all of this does not suffice to completely clarify the rejection of sexuality characteristic of hysteria in general, and of Dora's pathology in particular. We understand now why sexuality is linked to anxiety, but the actual disgust of sexuality still remains unexplained. One remembers Freud's idea that Dora's genital catarrh (leucorrhoea) is a symptom of masturbation. According to Freud, leucorrhea and hysterical symptoms are related: "…that in the case of hysterical patients suffering from leucorrhea any increase in the catarrh was regularly followed by an intensification of the hysterical symptoms, and especially loss of appetite and vomiting".[47] Although Freud does not exclude the gynecologists' conjecture that this connection might have an organic foundation, he gives preference to a psychological explanation.[48] Disorders of the genitals generate feelings of repugnance and disgust and lower the patient's self-esteem: "An abnormal secretion of the mucous membrane of the vagina is looked upon as a source of disgust".[49] Freud also reminds his readers of Dora's governess who

---

[45] Freud speaks in this context of 'somatic compliance'. The unconscious representation uses real somatic symptoms to express itself ("It cannot occur without the presence of a certain degree of somatic compliance offered by some normal or pathological process in or connected with one of the bodily organs"). Dora's cough for instance is not caused by the conversion of an unconscious representation into the body, but the representation uses the actual cough to express itself. It is soldered to it. As a result the cough doesn't disappear as it normally would. The predominance of the oral zone in Dora's pathology should also be regarded as a form of 'somatic compliance'. Freud, 'Fragment', p. 40, 52.
[46] Ibid., p. 80.
[47] Ibid., p. 83.
[48] Ibid., p. 84.
[49] Ibid.

taught her that all men are frivolous and untrustworthy. For Dora this must have meant, Freud intuits, that all men are like her father, frivolous and as therefore quite likely to suffer from a sexually transmitted infection. But Dora could only understand sexually transmitted infections on the basis of her own experience. Hence she equated a sexually transmitted infection with a disgusting discharge. The reconstruction of this unconscious reasoning finally allows Freud to understand the disgust that Dora felt at the moment Mr K. embraced her and she felt his erect penis: "Thus the disgust which was transferred on to the contact of the man would be a feeling which had been projected according to the primitive mechanism I have already mentioned, and would be related ultimately to her own leucorrhoea".[50]

Trauma and disposition

The *Three Essays* describe the hysterical disposition or, better still, the 'organic determinants' of hysteria. It would be incorrect to understand this disposition as the cause of the hysterical pathology. Although Freud is far from denying the hereditary aspects of psychopathology, he clearly defends a much more complex etiology of the neuroses.[51] We cannot discuss Freud's notion of disposition in too much detail here, but what I have argued so far allows me to shed some light on Freud's insights in this regard. I mentioned Freud's idea that the contamination of the sexual by the excremental constitutes a problem for every human being. But there is no direct, let alone causal link between this possibility and hysteria: "A knowledge of the paths does not render less necessary a knowledge of the forces which travel along them". Freud formulates a similar idea with regard to the *polymorphously perverse disposition*: "It is an instructive fact that under the influence of seduction, children can become polymorphously perverse, and can be tempted to all possible kinds of transgressions. This shows that the child already carries an appropriate aptitude within its disposition…".[52] In both cases the reference to a 'disposition' functions as a kind of necessary but not a sufficient condition for pathology and hysteria. We all bear the possibility of a contamination of the sexual by the excremental or of becoming polymorphously perverse. In some persons this possibility is more pronounced than in others. Even if the impact of accidental factors varies with the relative strength of the

---

[50] Ibid.
[51] Freud, *Three Essays (1905)*, pp. 84-86 (*SE 7*, pp. 235-236). Freud writes for instance: "In neurotics their sexual constitution, under which the effects of heredity are included, operates in combination with any accidental influences in their life which may disturb the development of normal sexuality". Ibid., pp. 50-51.
[52] Freud, *Three Essays*, p. 191.

dispositional factors, there are only few cases in which accidental factors are not a precondition for the realization of this possibility. This explains why Freud keeps referring to his seduction theory from 1895 throughout the 'Fragment'-text. He repeatedly insists that he did not give up this theory, but rather viewed it as incomplete.[53] Indeed, it had to be complemented by a theory of a *sexual constitution* with which the trauma interacts and which helps to explain its efficacy.[54] It is this interaction that the 'Fragment of an Analysis of a Case of Hysteria' exemplifies. The 'Fragment'-text explains why Dora could not overcome the possible contamination of the sexual by the excremental, as most of us do to a greater or lesser extent. This impossibility was all but inevitable; it depended on a *contingent* interaction between a disposition and accidental events and traumata.

Generalized seduction?

In Freud's view masturbation was a key factor in Dora's history. Masturbation is at the origin of Dora's leucorrhea and of her bed-wetting. Freud postulates a link between hysterical symptoms and masturbation.[55] He concludes: "Let it suffice if we can reach the conviction that in this case the occurrence of masturbation in childhood is established, and *that its occurrence cannot be an accidental element nor an immaterial one in the confirmation of the clinical picture*" (italics PvH).[56] Freud further claims that Dora stopped masturbating after overhearing her parents having sexual intercourse. He describes Dora's reaction in this context in purely mechanical terms: free-floating libido is automatically transformed into anxiety.

However, there are elements in Freud's description that allow for a different, less 'mechanical' approach. Dora cannot 'bind' the sexual excitation that is caused by overhearing her parents. Does this not mean that Dora was incapable, both affectively and intellectually, of understanding what happened to her at that very moment? Overhearing her parents is first and foremost a confrontation with adult sexuality for which she was not yet ready. We can interpret the sounds that come out of the room of Dora's parents as an enigmatic (sexual) message asking for a translation – a process that is bound to fail. I am of course thinking here of Laplanche's theory of generalized seduction that starts from the assumption of a fundamental asymmetry between the infant's experience

---

[53] Freud, 'Fragment', p. 27 – in note.
[54] Freud, 'My Views', p. 276. See also the introduction to this article.
[55] Freud, 'Fragment', p. 79.
[56] Ibid., p. 82.

of pleasure and adult sexuality.⁵⁷ The adult inevitably confronts the child with messages stemming from his or her unconscious that refer to a passionate, guilt-ridden, and orgasmic experience of sexuality. The small child is neither affectively nor physically prepared for these messages of the adult, mostly sent unknowingly. In Freud's terms, we would say that the child cannot bind them to adequate representations. According to Laplanche, this is why adult sexuality is essentially *enigmatic* for the little child.⁵⁸ The message confronts the child with a task of translation that it can only partially fulfill. Every effort for translation fails and leaves a leftover/remainder/vestigial experience that cannot be integrated in the child's psychic life. Sexuality thus becomes a 'foreign' element in its corporal and affective experience. By the same token, the confrontation with adult sexuality will have a *traumatic* character for the little child: the child is left at best with a partial response to something overwhelming with which it cannot adequately cope.⁵⁹

There are a number of places in the 'Fragment' that clearly point to this dimension of infantile sexual experience. I already mentioned the episode in which Dora overheard her parents talk about her father's syphilis and her aunt saying that he was 'already sick before their marriage'. Adult sexuality here inevitably appears as something threatening, something one should rightly fear. Her aunt's statement confronts Dora with a sexual message that she does not understand, even if she manages to relate it to 'indecent things' at a later stage. These 'indecent things', in her understanding at the time, bring sicknesses that can be transferred to others. Dora further links the threat of sexuality to the frivolous lifestyle of her father and men in general to whom she attributes sexually transmitted diseases. But she can only understand what these diseases are in terms of her own bodily experience, that is in analogy to her own loecorrhoea and hence as a disgusting discharge. Is it too risky a hypothesis then to say that Dora's disgust cannot be understood apart from the way in which she was confronted with adult sexuality as a child, and the way in which she managed (not) to translate it?

Conclusion

In publishing the 'Fragment of an Analysis of a Case of Hysteria', Freud wanted to prevent misunderstandings on his views on the relation between psychical

---

⁵⁷ J. Laplanche, *Nouveaux fondements pour la psychanalyse*. Paris: PUF (quadrige), 1987.
⁵⁸ Ibid., pp. 153-157.
⁵⁹ Ph. Van Haute, 'Humankind: A Sick Animal? On the Meaning and Importance of the Primacy of Sexuality in Freud, Fonagy, and Laplanche', in: *The Southern Journal of Philosophy, Tthe Spindel Supplement* 51 (2013), 4-16.

processes and organic determinants in hysteria. These 'organic determinants' constitute a sexual constitution or disposition that in principle should not be understood apart from accidental (traumatic) circumstances.[60] The hysterical disposition is fundamentally characterized by a contamination of the sexual by the excremental. Accordingly, understanding hysteria means first and foremost understanding how this contamination comes about. Freud explains that we all have to deal with the problematic relation between the sexual and excremental. Nobody escapes it. In this sense we all are to some extent hysteric.[61] But we still have to explain how this relation could become such a dramatic problem in Dora's case.

The traumatic events with Mr. K. that structure Freud's clinical exposition of Dora' life do not suffice to explain Dora's disgust for sexuality. This disgust is already presupposed, this is how the encounters with Mr K. can develop a traumatic meaning. Consider also the fact that Dora developed several hysterical symptoms before the first trauma with Mr K. Freud concludes from this that we should look for other, more original traumata in order to understand Dora's disgust and hysterical symptoms. One sees here the ambivalent and complex use of the term 'disposition' in Freud's text. Indeed, the Freudian disposition can itself not be thought apart from the traumatic events that shapes it. The relation between the sexual and the excremental is a problematic we all must deal with, but the actual contamination of the former by the latter – even if nobody completely escapes from it – can in most cases not be understood apart from accidental events. In terms of the 1915 edition of *Three Essays*, we could probably say that the disposition is constituted as "'a complemental series' in which the diminishing intensity of one factor is balanced by the increasing intensity of the other; there is, however, no reason to deny the existence of extreme cases at the two ends of the series".[62]

In his search for more fundamental events and traumata that could explain Dora's hysteria and dispositional disgust, Freud accords great importance to masturbation. He even goes as far as asking whether masturbation is not the determining cause of hysteria in general, Dora's *petite hystérie* in particular.[63] But the more important question here is why Dora stopped masturbating. This problematic brought us to the more general question as to the way in which Dora as a child was confronted with adult sexuality. Laplanche's theory of a generalized seduction allowed us to articulate the hypothesis that it is precisely this confrontation and Dora's answer to it that are at the basis of the

---

[60] Freud, *Three Essays*, p. 239; Freud, 'My Views'.
[61] Freud, *Three Essays*, p. 171.
[62] Ibid., p. 240.
[63] Freud, 'Fragment', pp. 81-82.

dispositional disgust explaining what Freud considers Dora's inconsistency in her relation to Mr K.[64]

My reading then shows the great importance of masturbation in Freud's text. This importance has very often been underestimated, probably because it is so unlikely for a contemporary reader that psychopathology would originate from masturbation. However, it also shows, more broadly, Freud's clinical genius. His text contains sufficient *clinical material* for a re-reading that turns it into a document illustrating the contemporary debates on Laplanche's generalized seduction and it's further development.

---

[64] This allows us to understand the following passage from the 1915 edition of the *Three Essays*: "We shall be in even closer harmony with psychoanalytic research if we give a place of preference among the accidental factors to the experiences of early childhood. The single aetiological series then falls into two, which may be called the dispositional and the definitive. In the first the constitution and the accidental experiences of childhood interact in the same manner as do the disposition and later traumatic experiences in the second". Freud, *Three Essays*, p. 240.

Sucking, Kissing and Disgust – Dora and the Theory of Infantile Sexuality

Herman Westerink

Though likely to be overshadowed by the grand groundbreaking texts Freud wrote and published in the period that coincides with the start and finish of the Dora case, the 'Fragment of an Analysis of a case of Hysteria' is a fascinating and important text. Its importance is not the least determined by its relation to the two major writings to which this case study is inherently linked. On the one hand there is *The Interpretation of Dreams* published some months before Freud started the treatment of the eighteen-year-old girl named Dora in October 1900. On the other hand there is the *Three Essays on the Theory of Sexuality* published in 1905 only shortly before the publication of the 'Fragment' in the *Monatsschrift für Psychiatrie und Neurologie* in November 1905. In this chapter I will first contextualize the Dora case, i.e., describe the relation of the case history with Freud's dream theory and studies in hysteria. Then, I will elaborate the significance of the Dora case for our reading of the 1905 edition of the *Three Essays*. I focus on three aspects in particular: the central place Freud assigns to sucking, kissing and disgust in his theory of infantile sexuality. My claim is that the 1905 theory of infantile sexuality can largely understood through and from Freud's analysis of Dora.

Dream and hysteria

The relation between *The Interpretation of Dreams* and the Dora case immediately becomes clear when we consider a letter to Wilhelm Fliess from January 1901. Freud writes:

> "I finished 'Dream and Hysteria' yesterday (…). It is a fragment of an analysis of a case of hysteria in which the explanations are grouped around two dreams; so it is really a continuation of the dream book".[1]

---

[1] *The Complete Letters of Sigmund Freud to Wilhelm Fliess* 1887–1904, J.M. Masson (Ed.). Cambridge, MA: The Belknap Press of Harvard University Press, 1985, p. 433.

This remark is confirmed by Freud in the prefatory remarks in the Dora case study. There Freud writes that the work "seemed to me peculiarly well-adapted for showing how dream-interpretation is woven into the history of a treatment and how it can become the means of filling in amnesia and elucidating symptoms".[2] Following this train of thought, the Dora case could indeed be read as an application of the theory of dream-interpretation in the clinical practice. The case study shows how the interpretation of dreams can contribute to psychoanalytic treatment – it shows the utilization of dream analysis. One might argue that this step was necessary due to the origins of *The Interpretation of Dreams* in Freud's self-analysis. After all, in the popular view on the development of Freudian theory, this self-analysis of dreams is often put forward as the source from which *The Interpretation of Dreams* was produced. However, this view can be contested. Despite the fact that part of the dream material was autobiographical, *The Interpretation of Dreams* was never simply the outcome of self-analysis. Freud had important theoretical arguments for engaging in the dream-project. In the Dora case he writes the following on this issue:

> "I must once more insist, just as I did on that time, that a thorough investigation of the problems of dreams is an indispensable prerequisite for any comprehension of the mental processes in hysteria and the other psychoneuroses."[3]

In other words, the project of the analysis of dreams was from the start embedded in his studies on hysteria in particular and the psychoneuroses in general. In the Dora case Freud is explicit about what he hoped to gain from the dream-analysis. He writes:

> "the dream is one of the roads along which consciousness can be reached by the psychical material which, on account of the opposition aroused by its content, has been cut off from consciousness and repressed, and has thus become pathogenic. The dream, in short, is one of the *détours by which repression can be evaded*."[4]

---

[2] S. Freud, 'Fragment of an Analysis of a Case of Hysteria' (1905 [1901]), *SE* 7, p. 10.
[3] Ibid., p. 11.
[4] Ibid., 15.

In *The Interpretation of Dreams* we find similar statements: the dream-analysis is a way to trace a pathological idea back through a chain of memories to its source. The dream then has the status of a symptom amongst the other symptoms of the psychoneuroses, in particular of hysteria.[5] In several texts from the late 1890s Freud had already noticed the significance of the dream as a symptom in hysteria – the dream here closely resembling hysterical hallucinations. According to Freud, the fact that there were strong analogies between the dream and certain pathological mechanisms (such as condensation, compromise formation and associations with disregard of contradictions) in the psychoneuroses implied that dream-analysis gained clinical importance.[6] Here, the idea already present in Freud's earlier writings of a continuum between pathology and normality proved to work in two directions: not only could the psychopathologies inform about aspects of general human nature (such as unconscious motives, representations and affects, memories, repression, resistance, and et cetera), but also aspects of normal life – such as dreams (or also jokes) – could shed light on pathological phenomena and mechanisms involved in neurotic symptom formation. Seen from this perspective, the Dora case was not about showing the clinical utilization of the fruits of self-analysis, but was actually meant to bring in a further synthesis the earlier ideas on the mechanisms and unconscious dynamics involved in hysteria and dreams. This implies that the 'Fragment' is not only the continuation of the dream book, but also of Freud's writings on hysteria in particular from the 1890s. The original title of the Dora case, 'Dream and Hysteria', in fact perfectly expresses this purpose. Freud confirms this in the opening sentences of his text – he intends to substantiate "certain views upon the pathogenesis of hysterical symptoms and upon the mental processes occurring in hysteria" as presented in *Studies on Hysteria* from 1895 and 'The Aetiology of Hysteria' from 1896.

At this point we need to ask the question why Freud found it necessary to postpone the publication of the case study – which was as good as finished in the Spring of 1901 – until 1905? Why wait four years with showing the clinical utilization of the dream-analysis? An answer to these questions is not just a matter of speculation. In a letter to Fliess from 1901 we find an indication of a possible answer. Freud writes:

---

[5] S. Freud, *The Interpretation of Dreams* (1900), *SE* 4, pp. 100-101.
[6] S. Freud, *The Interpretation of Dreams*, *SE* 5, p. 597. Compare 'Draft L '(1897) on the architecture of hysteria, phantasy and dreams, and section 20 on dream-analysis of the 'Project for a Scientific Psychology' (1895), in: S. Freud, 'Extracts from the Fliess Papers', *SE* 1, pp. 248-249, 338-341.

> "'Dreams and Hysteria' should not disappoint you, so far as it goes. The chief thing in it is again psychology, the utilization of dreams, and a few peculiarities of unconscious mental activity. There are only *glimpses* of the organic background – in connection with the erotogenic zones and bisexuality. But bisexuality is mentioned and specifically recognized once and for all, and the ground is prepared for detailed treatment of it on another occasion."[7]

What Freud calls 'glimpses of the organic side – the erotogenic zones and bisexuality' will be central issues in the *Three Essays*. We could therefore read the cited letter as follows: Freud felt comfortable with the 'Fragment' in as far as it dealt with Dora's dreams, however, his ideas "about the infantile germs of perversion, about the erotogenic zones, and about our predisposition towards bisexuality" were hardly developed in 1901.[8] The 'Fragment' indeed was a fragment because substantial theoretical ground was still missing. There were merely 'glimpses' of what would become the more full-fledged theory of infantile sexuality in 1905. For example, in the 'Fragment' Freud highlights the mouth "as a primary 'erotogenic zone'" in Dora's sexual life,[9] but it is not without reason that he puts erotogenic zones between quotation marks: in Dora we do not find any theory or definition of the erotogenic zones. Another example is Freud's remarks on the perversions as being "contained in the undifferentiated sexual disposition of the child".[10] This statement points forward to the notion of the polymorphous-perverse nature of the sexual drive as characterizing the human sexual disposition. Still, this theory is far from fully developed in 1901 – during that period the notion of the drive had not yet even been properly introduced into Freud's vocabulary. In regards to the perversions, it was in the Dora case that Freud articulated what was then further developed in the *Three Essays*, namely that the perversions "are contained in the undifferentiated sexual disposition of the child" which means that the later actual perversions are not bestial or degenerate, but remainders of a general human sexual disposition.[11] Freud in his previous writings had seldom elaborated perversion, and if so, he was inclined to view it analogously to the popular view in his days: perversions were first of all immoral sexual activities. It is telling that Freud in his early writings does not seem to make the principal distinction between *perversions*

---

[7] *The Complete Letters of Freud to Fliess*, pp. 434-436.
[8] Freud, 'Fragment', pp. 113-114. The quotation is from the 1905 'Postscript' to the Dora case.
[9] Ibid., p. 52.
[10] Ibid., p. 50.
[11] Ibid.

(the sexual activities that do not correspond with the purpose of nature, i.e., propagation) and *perversities* (incidental immoral sexual activities) one does find in Krafft-Ebing's *Psychopathia sexualis*.[12] And as regards bisexuality – a term Freud took from Fliess – it is shortly after finishing the case history in 1901 that Freud writes to Fliess about his new project: a book on *Die menschliche Bisexualität* exploring not so much the anatomical-biological part Fliess seemed to have been more interested in, but the psychic aspect of bisexuality, i.e., the (at least) two conflicting sexual impulses from which the notion of repression could probably be explained.[13] It was Dora's random switching between male and female orientations and male and female objects that had given impetus to the study of this subject.

At the same time one could argue from reading the letters to Fliess that it was the central intuitions from the analysis of Dora that would develop into the theory of infantile sexuality in the *Three Essays*. It was the treatment of Dora that provided Freud the building blocks for a more systematic reflection on sexuality. This is apparent not only given the centrality of the aforementioned intuitions on the infantile germs of perversion, the erotogenic zones, and the predisposition towards bisexuality. Two other central aspects of the *Three Essays* underscore the close relation between the Dora case and the theory of infantile sexuality. Firstly, there is the fact that Freud takes hysteria as a model for the study of sexuality – and the Dora case presents the theory of hysteria at that moment. And secondly, there are the interrelated phenomena of sensual sucking (*lutschen*), kissing and disgust first explored in the Dora case that are at the core of Freud's depiction of infantile sexuality. The rest of the book chapter is devoted to the exploration of these two issues.

Dora as model for the theory of infantile sexuality

In the *Three Essays* Freud approaches human sexuality, and more specifically infantile sexuality, from the perspective of hysteria.[14] Why start from the perspective of hysteria? A first answer to this question would be to say that

---

[12] For example in Draft K from January 1896 Freud speaks of *Perversitäten* (instead of *Perversionen*) relative to the emergence of the neuroses. *The Complete Letters of Freud to Fliess*, pp. 162-169, p. 163.
On Krafft-Ebing and the distinction between perversion and perversity see, Ph. Van Haute & H. Westerink, 'De perversie en de terugkeer van het kwade', in: S. Freud, *Drie verhandelingen over de theorie van de seksualiteit (1905)*, Ph. Van Haute & H. Westerink (Eds.). Nijmegen: Vantilt, 2017, pp. 131-155.
[13] *The Complete Letters of Freud to Fliess*, p. 448.
[14] S. Freud, *Three Essays on the Theory of Sexuality. The 1905 Edition*, Ph. Van Haute, U. Kistner & H. Westerink (Eds.). London/New York: Verso, 2016, pp. 23ff (*SE* 7, pp. 163ff).

the starting point is self-evident; Freud's psychoanalytic practice and theories were thus far largely based on the study of hysteria. Why choose a starting point other than one's own primal expertise? But in fact, studying sexuality from the perspective of hysteria, or for that matter from the psychoneuroses, was far from self-evident. The crucial discovery that made this possible was Freud's questioning of the status of accidental factors in the aetiology of the psychoneuroses. His theories on the aetiology of hysteria from the mid 1890s were largely built on the notion of 'abnormal' traumatic sexual experiences in childhood. In the *Three Essays* and more explicitly also in 'My Views on the Part played by Sexuality in the Aetiology of the Neuroses' from 1906, Freud argues both that this theory could remain intact, but that even so the accidental factors could no longer be held decisive in the aetiology of all psychoneuroses. A first argument that leads Freud to this conclusion was the role played by phantasy in the formation of neurotic symptoms. The analysis of Dora had substantiated this conclusion: Dora's spasmodic cough is interpreted by Freud as the symptom of a pubertal phantasy of fellatio she finds highly repulsive and subsequently represses.[15] The prerequisite for this phantasy was not some infantile sexual experience involving an adult person, but was of a somatic nature: Dora had been an enthusiastic *Lutscherin* – sensual sucker – indicating that her "mouth is to be regarded as a primary 'erotogenic zone'".[16] According to Freud, the hysterical symptom could not occur without the participation of the erotogenic zone. Freud writes: "[the hysterical symptom] cannot occur without the presence of a certain degree of *somatic compliance* offered by some normal or pathological process in or connected with one of the bodily organs".[17] In the case of Dora her intense activity of the mouth at an early age "determines the subsequent presence of a somatic compliance on the part of the tract of mucous membrane which begins at the lips".[18] The conclusion Freud draws from this in in 'My Views' is that the importance of "the factors of constitution and heredity necessarily gained the upper-hand once more".[19] He immediately adds that this does not mean a return to those predecessors in neurology, psychiatry and sexology that were inclined to explain the psychoneuroses from an abnormal neuropathic disposition. It means that the 'somatic compliance' and the significance of specific erotogenic zones should be related to a general

---

[15] Freud, 'Fragment', p. 51.
[16] Ibid., 52.
[17] Ibid., 40.
[18] Ibid., 52.
[19] S. Freud, 'My Views on the Part played by Sexuality in the Aetiology of the Neuroses' (1906), *SE* 7, p. 275.

human sexual disposition. The case of Dora had convinced Freud that the study of the psychoneuroses was impossible without reference to and hence insight in this general human sexual disposition.

But then again, how to study this disposition? Freud's answer is 'through the study of hysteria'. The reference to the sexual disposition called for a redefinition of the relation between pathology and normality. As already briefly mentioned above, Freud introduced the idea that psychopathologies, notably hysteria, can be seen as exaggerations and intensifications of normal sexual impulses and acts. In hysteria we find constitutionally higher-than-average sexual energy and simultaneously we find repression of sexual impulses in excess of the normal measure. Hence, hysteria is a pathology at least close to normality, Freud claims, and at the same time it is characterized by higher-than-average quantities of sexual energy, by intensified and excessive repression and by corporeal symptom formations that appear to be magnifications and caricatures of normal corporeal expressions of the human emotional life.[20] For these reasons hysteria presents itself as suitable for an anthropological approach to sexuality and hence to human nature as such.[21]

What then can be said to be the building blocks of human sexuality when this is enquired from the perspective of hysteria (and its negative, the perversions)? Some of the elements have already been mentioned: the issue of bisexuality and the relation between hysteria and perversions (the similar content of hysteric unconscious phantasies and pervert actions; the fact that erogenous zones and hysterogenic zones are identical). The Dora case also provides other important intuitions and insights. According to Freud, Dora's first reaction to Herr K.'s seductions – at the age of fourteen Dora is kissed on the mouth by Herr K., an occasion at which she also feels the pressure of his erect member against her body – shows that she was already completely hysterical. That is to say, the occasion for sexual excitement elicited strong feelings of unpleasure – of disgust, more concretely. It is this disgust as the symptom of repression in the erotogenic oral zone that points towards the organization of Dora's sexuality in childhood. Freud argues that the disgust was originally a reaction to the smell of excrement that in early childhood is easily associated with the genitals and their function of micturition (not their reproductive function which is after

---

[20] Freud, *Three Essays*, pp. 23-25 (*SE* 7, pp. 163-164).
[21] See also, Ph. Van Haute & T. Geyskens, *A Non-Oedipal Psychoanalysis? A Clinical Anthropology of Hysteria in the Work of Freud and Lacan*. Leuven: Leuven University Press, 2012; Ph. Van Haute & H. Westerink, 'Hysteria, Sexuality, and the Deconstruction of Normativity. Re-reading Freud's 1905 edition of *Three Essays on the Theory of Sexuality*', in: S. Freud, *Three Essays on the Theory of Sexuality. The 1905 Edition*, xiii-lxxvi.

all unknown to the child).²² As the case of Little Hans from 1909 will later confirm, the male and female genitals are primarily seen as widdlers – an organ for discharge of urine.²³

In other words, from Dora Freud learns that in infantile sexuality we can find the association of sexuality with the excremental – an association that in hysteria (of an adult) is not overcome, but actually a constant threat. The hysteric constantly fears the contamination of sexuality (sexual pleasure and excitement) by the excremental (smell – unpleasure – disgust).²⁴ A specific factor in Dora's puberty contributed to this: Dora suffered a catarrh (leucorrhoea) that caused foul-smelling vaginal discharge. Dora interpreted her catarrh as a venereal disease she had 'inherited' from her father. According to Freud, the kissing scene with Herr K. pressing his member against Dora's body showed that Dora's reaction of intense disgust to the contact with Herr K.'s erect member was related to her immediate association with disgusting discharge.²⁵

In the Dora case Freud thus gained insight in two issues that were also elaborated in the theory of infantile sexuality. Firstly, the hysteric patient shows in an exaggerated manner a contradiction found in general human sexuality, namely "a sexual rejection taken too far on the one hand, and an excessively felt sexual need, on the other".²⁶ Secondly, Freud recognized the importance of the spontaneous disgust as reaction to sexual pleasure and excitement. In *Three Essays* Freud argues that this spontaneous disgust is paradigmatic of the more general fact that sexual pleasure can turn into unpleasure without the

---

²² Freud, 'Fragment', pp. 28ff.
²³ On Little Hans see, T. Geyskens, *Our Original Scenes. Freud's Theory of Sexuality*. Leuven, Leuven University Press, 2005, pp. 29-34. Contrary to Dora, Hans is not hysteric, i.e., the little boy is fascinated by widdlers, which are central in his infantile world view, but clearly without any sign of a threat of contamination of the oral zone (which is not central in Hans' infantile sexuality), hence, without the experience of disgust. Instead, there is another threat, namely the threat of losing the widdler.
²⁴ How exactly this unpleasure is triggered, Freud does not tell. Somehow there is a 'contamination' with something that smells bad, i.e., anal and/or genital discharge, resulting the first response, namely to gag. Is it indeed the unpleasurable smell of excrements that interferes with the sensual sucking? Or is it perhaps the spitting up of milk by babies that is first experienced as pleasurable and – like other excretions – valued as parts of one's body, but that likely will evoke disgust since the infant is unable to make a distinction between oral, anal and genital discharge? The second theoretical option connects to what Freud writes on excrements and excretion in the 1916-1917 'Introductory Lectures on Psycho-Analysis' (1916), *SE* 16, pp. 314-315.
²⁵ Freud, 'Fragment', pp. 75-76, 84. See also, Ph. Van Haute & T. Geyskens, *A Non-Oedipal Psychoanalysis? A Clinical Anthropology of Hysteria in the Works of Freud and Lacan*. Leuven, Leuven University Press, 2012, p. 48.
²⁶ Freud, *Three Essays*, p. 25 (*SE* 7, p. 165).

interference of an external factor (an experience, norm, or principle). Such unpleasure should, however, also not be interpreted as a natural 'instinctual' rejection of the 'foul' or the 'bad': the perversions give evidence that there is not a predetermined innate response to the excremental.[27] Freud therefore introduces a notion he calls "organically conditioned" reaction formations.[28] A year later Freud will refer to these reaction formations as "organic sexual repression" indicating that infantile sexuality could be described in terms of purely physiological processes.[29] Disgust was not the result of predetermined actions or ideas about whatever one might consider the disgusting; disgust means to gag (being unable to swallow and about to vomit) over the (smell of the) excremental, i.e., over the discharge.

Another important lesson Freud learnt from the analysis of Dora was that the sexual object relations and phantasies of seduction very much belong to the realm of pubertal and adult sexual life. In the Dora case we find that Freud indeed refers hereditary factors, the sexual disposition, the erotogenic zones and organically conditioned processes when dealing with sexuality in childhood. In the *Three Essays* these findings are confirmed in a theory in which infantile sexuality is "without an object, that is, *autoerotic*".[30] Infantile sexuality is nothing but a physical-pleasurable activity originating from the sexual drive and the excitability of erogenous zones. Also, the case of Dora revealed that there was no primacy of the genital zone: the predominant erotogenic zone in Dora's childhood was the oral zone. And it is this zone that will be the starting point for Freud's depiction of infantile sexuality.

Sensual sucking

In the *Three Essays* Freud does not present a clear-cut definition of infantile sexuality. His approach is more descriptive and indirect. He writes: "For reasons which will appear later, I shall take sensual sucking (sucking blissfully) as a model of the infantile sexual manifestations."[31] Why does Freud take sensual

---

[27] Freud will basically argue that the fact that humans started to walk upright and thus estranged from earthly dirt and bad smells, made it possible to experience disgust – as opposed to animals who do not experience disgust. In other words, from the perspective of the natural instincts in animal life there is no evidence for a natural reaction against the excremental. On this issue see Ph. Van Haute & T. Geyskens, *Confusion of Tongues: The Primacy of Sexuality in Freud, Ferenczi and Laplanche*. New York, Other Press, 2004, pp. 44–45.
[28] Freud, *Three Essays*, p. 39 (*SE 7*, p. 177). On this issue see, Ph. Van Haute & H. Westerink, 'Hysteria, Sexuality, and the Deconstruction of Normativity', xxix-xxxiv.
[29] Freud, 'My Views', p. 278.
[30] Freud, *Three Essays*, p. 82 (*SE 7*, p. 233).
[31] Freud, *Three Essays*, p. 40 (*SE 7*, p. 179).

sucking as a model? Let us resume what Freud learned from Dora: Dora's pubertal phantasies show precisely the same content as the actions of perverts; Dora's symptoms point towards the oral zone as the primal erotogenic zone, which is confirmed by the fact that she was a *Lutscherin* who found sexual self-gratification by sucking; the perversions can be traced back to the undifferentiated sexual disposition of the child. Freud adds that not only Dora but also other hysteric patients provided accounts of such self-gratification by sucking.[32] In other words, Freud argues that it is Dora and the anonymous other hysteric patients that point toward the sexual nature of infantile sucking. The obvious question is then: What does Freud mean by 'sexual' if the model is infantile sensual sucking? At this point, the reference to Krafft-Ebing's *Psychoapathia Sexualis* in the Dora case and the more implicit discussion with Krafft-Ebing on the perversions in the *Three Essays* is important.[33] This reference does not simply identify Krafft-Ebing with the opponents that held perversions to be bestial or degenerate. This reference much more shows the underlying issue at stake. For, according to Krafft-Ebing and others (such as Albert Moll), sexuality should be defined in purely functional terms from a Darwinian perspective, i.e., pubertal and adult sexuality as the manifestation a genital drive (*Geschlechtstrieb*) that is grounded in a reproduction instinct in the service of the preservation of the species, which implied the normal (natural) choice of sexual object, the heterosexual partner. From this perspective sexuality was analogous to hunger as the expression of the need for ingestion in the service of self-preservation. It was this view of sexuality that determined the identification of what Krafft-Ebing called "the anomalies in the sexual function",[34] i.e. the sexual perversions that proved to be deviation from the functional norm. In this way, Krafft-Ebing could list the perversions: sadism, masochism, fetishism, and inversion. Dora in particular had shown the way towards a position that completely turned the opinion of his predecessors upside down: the sexual disposition did not first manifest itself in the genital-reproductive drive in puberty, but in the infantile polymorphous-perverse autoeroticism that could be witnessed in Dora's self-gratification by sucking. Taking sensual sucking as a model thus marked Freud's critique of the model of his predecessors.

---

[32] Freud, 'Fragment', p. 51.
[33] Ibid., p. 50; Freud, *Three Essays*, first part. On Krafft-Ebing and Freud see, H. Oosterhuis, *Stepchildren of Nature: Krafft-Ebing, Psychiatry, and the Making of Sexual Identity*. Chicago: University of Chicago Press, 2000; Ph. Van Haute & H. Westerink (Eds.), *Deconstructing Normativity? Re-reading Freud's 1905 Three Essays*. London/New York: Routledge, 2017.
[34] R. von Krafft-Ebing, *Psychopathia Sexualis, with Especial Reference to the Antipathic Sexual Instinct: A Medico-Forensic Study*, F.E. Klaf (Ed.). New York: Arcade Publishing, 1965, p. 32.

However, Freud also remains close to the Darwinian background: the sexual drive should be considered "analogous to the desire for food, that is, to hunger".[35] But these two do no longer relate to each other in terms of 'preservation'. Freud develops another relation between the two. The desire for food is still indeed the expression of an instinct (*Trieb*) for self-preservation. According to Feud, the actual food intake does not only result in the satisfaction of this nutrition drive (full stomach), but also produces a side effect that Freud defines as 'sexual'. While sucking the mother's breast – or a milk bottle as a matter of fact – "the child's lips, in our view, behaved like an erogenous zone, presumably the stimulation by the warm flow of milk was the cause of the pleasurable sensation".[36] The food intake produces a pleasurable sensation at the lips and in the mouth, and it is this sensation that the child seeks to reproduce in every act of rhythmic sensual sucking. According to Freud, the paradigm for infantile sexuality is the lips kissing themselves. On this he writes:

> "The child does not make use of an extraneous body for sucking, but prefers a part of its own skin because it is more convenient, because it makes it independent of the external world, which it is not yet able to control, and because in that way it provides itself, as it were, with a second erogenous zone [the skin], albeit of an inferior kind. The inferiority of this second zone is among the reasons why at a later date the child seeks the corresponding parts – the lips – of another person. ("It's a pity I can't kiss myself," the child seems to be saying.)"[37]

From all this we can understand how Freud understands infantile sexuality. It is strictly autoerotic pleasure, first discovered at but then also detached from the food intake. It is non-intersubjective and not phantasmatical. It is a pleasurable sensation that the child and later also the adult will seek to reproduce, first, at one's own body (sensual sucking), later in the context of the organization of pubertal and adult sexuality through and in object relations (kissing).

According to Freud, those children that strongly engage in sensual sucking will later, as adults, "become gourmets in kissing, will be inclined to perverse kissing, or, if males, will have a powerful motive for drinking and smoking. If however, the repression ensues, they will feel disgust at food and produce

---

[35] Freud, *Three Essays*, p. 1 (*SE* 7, p. 135).
[36] Ibid., p. 42 (*SE* 7, p. 181).
[37] Ibid., pp. 42-43 (*SE* 7, p. 182).

hysterical vomiting".[38] Freud adds a reference to "women patients" suffering from eating disorders, throat problems and vomiting – in short, the kind of symptoms found in the Dora case. We find here an illustration of the idea that 'hysteria is the negative of the perversion': the 'perverse' infantile activity of sensual sucking can either be continued in adult sexual life and been brought into culture or it can be repressed – when associated with the excremental (discharge) – and produce hysterical symptoms.

As regards the vicissitudes of sensual sucking that are not repressed, there are actually two options. On the one hand, the 'perverse' infantile sensual sucking can be continued as 'positive' perversion in an adult sexual life exclusively fixated on sexual acts that (from the perspective of infantile sexuality) are in continuity with primacy of a specific erogenous zone, and that (in context of the normal, conventional organization of adult sexuality) do not serve the purpose of reproduction. One could think here of activities such as fellatio or the licking of shit that, according to Freud, are clearly perverse and – in the latter case – also evidently pathological. On the other hand, there is the process of sublimation by which "excessively strong excitations arising from particular sources of sexuality finds an outlet by making them useful in other fields".[39] Freud's references to artistic creativity and other cultural achievements are hardly helpful to understand what is meant here when we think of the case of sensual sucking and the primacy of the oral zone. Freud, however, does give us another clue as to what the third option consists of — something between perversion (fixation and exclusiveness) and hysteria (repression). On this issue Freud writes the following:

> "In so far as the perverse actions are inserted in the performance of the normal sexual act as preparatory or intensifying contributions, they are in reality not perversions at all. The gulf between normal and perverse sexuality is of course very much narrowed by facts of this kind. It is an easy conclusion that normal sexuality has emerged out of something that was in existence before it, by weeding out certain features of that material as unserviceable and collecting together the rest in order to subordinate them to a new aim, that of reproduction."[40]

Although these lines were written down almost a decade after the publication of the *Three Essays*, they express perfectly what Freud was hinting at already

---

[38] Ibid., p. 43 (*SE* 7, p. 182).
[39] Ibid., p. 87 (*SE* 7, p. 238).
[40] Freud, 'Introductory Lectures', p. 322.

in 1905. Infantile 'perverse' sexual activities such as sensual sucking can be continued in adult sexual life as part of — that is to say, subordinate to — the normal sexual life wherein disgust at the partner's erogenous zones, smells, and discharges is at least partly overcome. It is exactly because the normal adult sexual life cannot be reduced to the reproductive function[41] that kissing is held in great esteem in most cultures. In other words, it is exactly by integrating 'perverse' pleasurable sexual activities into the organization of adult sexual life that the normal sexual life becomes possible. Without the (generally human) tendency to reproduce the pleasurable sensations experienced in childhood there is no adult sexual life. All of this can be illustrated in the example of kissing.

Kissing and the overcoming of disgust

Under the heading 'Deviations in Respect of the Sexual Aim', Freud writes:

> "What is regarded as normal sexual aim [the actions impelled by the drive] is the union of the genitals in the act known as copulation, which dissolves sexual tension and temporarily extinguishes the sexual drive in a satisfaction analogous to the sating of hunger."[42]

According to Freud, this is the 'popular view' represented in the academic literature by scholars such as Krafft-Ebing and Moll. This view, however, cannot be maintained given the fact that in every normal sexual process perverse elements are involved. For example, in every normal adult sexual life there is not only copulation, but also the touching of and gazing at the other person's body – activities that are accompanied by pleasure and contributing to excitation. Given the fact that Freud takes sensual sucking as model for understanding infantile sexuality, it comes as no surprise that already here Freud is particularly interested in the phenomenon of kissing:

> "The kiss, one particular contact of this kind, between the mucous membrane of the lips of the two persons concerned, has attained a high sexual value among many cultures (including the most highly developed ones), although the parts of the body involved do not belong to the genital apparatus but form the entrance to the digestive tract."[43]

---

[41] In that hypothetical case a marriage, for example, would be nothing but a functional contract between two heterosexual partners that want to preserve the species.
[42] Freud, *Three Essays*, pp. 12-13 (*SE* 7, p. 149).
[43] Ibid., p. 13 (*SE* 7, p. 150).

From the perspective of the popular view, kissing would have to be considered a perverse activity, and Freud indeed confirms this later when he writes: "Even a kiss can claim to be described as a perverse act, since it consists in the bringing together of two oral erotogenic zones instead of the two genitals".[44] We have already established that kissing should be understood as the adult sexual activity that seeks to reproduce the pleasure experienced in infantile sensual sucking. As a perverse activity it is thus perfectly in line with the polymorphous perverse nature of infantile sexuality. At this point Freud points at an interesting issue that connects to our previous discussion of the fact that some perverse activities can be integrated in normal sexual life. Kissing is not simply a continuation of infantile activities. Like other infantile sexual activities, the pleasure experienced in sensual sucking in most cases will effect unpleasure, i.e., disgust. This reaction formation is after all not confined to the lives of hysterics. Following this line of reasoning, one might expect that in adult sexual life kissing results the same feeling of disgust as for example the use of the other person's toothbrush. However, this is clearly not the case, says Freud, which shows us that the disgust is "purely conventional".[45] The question is how this relates to the disgust as a form of organic conditioned reaction formations.

In order to answer this question we must first look at the way the cultural (moral, religious) conventions relate to the reaction formations. According to Freud, the reaction formations such as disgust and shame – but probably also anxiety as a reaction against rage[46] – are psychic counter-forces that are spontaneously constructed in order to repress the unpleasure that somehow results from sexual excitation. That means, that disgust cannot be seen as the earliest manifestation of internalized cultural morality, and also not as the result of an interaction with the external world. Disgust is not, for example, the effect of intersubjectivity, of some kind of response to an object. The relation between the organically conditioned limitation to excitation and cultural morality is actually the other way around. Cultural morality can only follow and impress "somewhat more clearly and deeply" the psychic lines "previously drawn organically."[47] In other words, cultural morality (laws, prohibitions, norms, but of course also conventions) can only be interiorized when connecting to basic psychic patterns and dams that are already in place – and if these patterns are not in place, cultural morality will be easily dismissed. Moral conventions thus follow and strengthen organic processes. This model also implies that there is

---

[44] Freud, 'Introductory Lectures', p. 322.
[45] Freud, *Three Essays*, p. 14 (*SE* 7, p. 151).
[46] See, H. Westerink, 'Der problematische Ort der Wut im Denken Freuds über Aggression', in: *Zeitschrift: texte* 36 (2017/4), pp. 27-46.
[47] Freud, *Three Essays*, p. 39 (*SE* 7, p. 178).

no natural innate norm for distinguishing between normal and perverse sexual activities – the reaction formations are not actualizations of an already present innate norm, but indeed spontaneous reactions relative to sexual excitation. The exact architecture and strength of the 'patterns and dams' thus vary from person to person.

Freud's critique of a cultural morality expressing a 'natural' distinction between normal sexuality and perversion, leaves no alternative but to say that morality is a matter of convention and consensus. Having said this, we still need to answer the question how the reaction formation relates to cultural morality. From what we have said, we can conclude that cultural morality is not simply repressive. In his later writings, when aggression becomes the more central problem, Freud will very strongly stress the opposition between the individual's drives and culture's demand for repression and renunciation. Even in 1908 in his text '"Civilized" Sexual Ethics and Modern Nervous Disease' the view on cultural morality is already clearly marked by the notion of repression and prohibition.[48] But in his earlier writings the theory is different. The fact that kissing could easily be considered disgusting, but is actually held in great esteem, points in very different direction: the cultural conventions may actually nuance the reaction formations, giving room to the experience of sexual pleasure by putting certain 'perverse' activities in the service of the genital drive. Through functionalization of sexual activities, looking at, touching and kissing another person's body can be experienced as pleasurable – to a certain extent the conventions thus nuance the limits previously drawn organically. To conclude, disgust is a convention in as far the cultural morality does not only follow the psychic reaction formations, but actually may follow and impress some psychic lines more deeply and clearly than others.

Freud's important, but hardly systematically elaborated, thoughts on the relation between reaction formation and cultural morality are an important part of the 1905 theory of sexuality that is focused on the importance of sexual constitution and the vicissitudes of the variety of sexual pleasures, needs, excitations, activities and objects in both infantile and later in adult life. The repressive character of cultural morality is not put to the fore, contrary to many of his writings on culture (and religion). Again, the Dora case is likely to have been of great importance here. Despite the decorum of the case – a bourgeois Viennese family life – cultural morality does not play a major role in the case history. The constitutional aspects are decisive, and on this Freud writes:

---

[48] Freud, '"Civilized" Sexual Ethics and Modern Nervous Disease' (1908), *SE* 9.

"For if Dora felt unable to yield to her love for the man [Herr K.], if in the end she repressed that love instead of surrendering to it, there was no factor upon which her decision depended more directly than upon her premature sexual enjoyment and its consequence – her bed-wetting, her catarrh, her disgust."[49]

Having referred here to this problem, which can be identified as the dynamics of excitation and reaction formation, Freud immediately adds that these constitutional determinants can later (in puberty and adulthood) result in different kinds of behavior. And it is here, where cultural morality connects to constitutional patterns, that Dora's 'intellectual and moral upbringing' becomes decisive. This aspect of the Dora case also helps to us understand Freud's train of thought in the *Three Essays*.

---

[49] Freud, 'Fragment', p. 87.

Dora, the Un-Ending and ever Unraveling Story

Jeanne Wolff Bernstein

The case of Dora does not cease to fascinate the post-Freudian generations and continues to evoke various debates about her treatment, her sexuality and her symptomatology. Readers, students and analysts alike are at the same time puzzled by Freud's grave omissions and errors in his treatment of Dora and astonished by his equally brilliant insights into the workings of dreams and symptoms. It may be argued that Freud tried to accomplish too much in this case, attempting to turn it into a show case about the workings of dreams and the internal dynamics of hysteria, as the initial title of this text was supposed to be 'Dream and Hysteria'[1] before Freud entitled it 'A Fragment Of An Analysis of A Case of Hysteria'. 'Fragment', however, is a somewhat unfortunate translation of the German title 'Bruchstück einer Hysterie-Analyse', because 'Bruchstück' unlike 'fragment' carries the notion of a 'break' inside itself. With the case of Dora, we are not only given a 'piece' of an analysis, but we are also made to witness a 'break' in an analytic treatment and a paradigmatic break from previous ideas that Freud had developed which he never really re-integrated into the case of Dora. I think that the various books and plays which have been published about Dora, such as *Dora, A Case of Hysteria* by the Playwrights Guild of Canada (1994) or the musical *Dora* by Mainstreet Musicals by Larry Botniker or Deborah Levy's dramatization of Dora for the BBC comprise attempts to understand and confront this curious analytic and theoretical break.

Dora, the pirouette and accomplice of numerous intrigues

Dora could not and cannot be laid to rest. The case, I believe, troubled Freud a great deal, not only the re-naming of the case and the delayed publication of its text serves as evidence of his grand hesitation to bring this case to the public eye, but also his return to the case in 1923, proves how much he was still haunted by Dora and the mis-handling and mis-understanding of her case. 1923 constitutes an interesting year for Freud, since it is not just the year of the grand work *The Id and the Ego,* but also the year, he feels compelled to go back to two important texts of 1905, namely the case of Dora and *The Three Essays*

---

[1] S. Freud, 'A Fragment of An Analysis of A Case of Hysteria' (1905 [1901]), *SE* 7, p. 10.

of Sexuality.[2] During that year, he undertakes important corrections about his theory of sexuality and admits his oversight of the importance of transference in the case of Dora.[3] In addition, I want to argue that the Dora case cannot be understood without a retroactive reading of 'The Psychogenesis of a Case of Homosexuality in a Woman' which Freud published without much reservation and hesitation in 1920, twenty years after Dora dismissed him and went about her ways. I am not the first one to notice the curious cross-sections between the Dora case, 'The Psychogenesis of a Case of Homosexuality in a Woman' and Freud's own daughter Anna whose lesbian tendencies became more evident to Freud, in the early twenties.[4]

Unlike Freud's self-avowed statement that he names things, particularly, sexual matters, by their name – "J'appelle un chat un chat"[5] –, the construction of Dora's case is not a case "of speaking about things in a dry and direct matter"[6] but an instance of intrigues, double crossings, omissions, betrayals, conflicted heterosexual and homosexual desires and lost voices, Dora's, in particular and Freud's own more reasonable and modest voice as well. The voice of the young collaborator with Josef Breuer of *Studies of Hysteria* (1895) and the thoughtful, inquisitive and learned voice of *The Interpretation of Dreams* (1900) has vanished and been exchanged for a more brash, seemingly self-assured voice which wishes to demonstrate with bravado the "intimate structure of a neurotic disorder and the determination of its symptoms"[7] and to show at the same time, the originality of his dream analysis technique. Freud appears to be blinded by his strong identification with Mr K. (Herr Zellenka, whose sister he had already treated and whom he may have known from vacations spent in the same resort town as the Zellenkas and Bauers, i.e. Merano) when he attempts to prove beyond any single doubt that repressed sexual wishes and desires resided behind

---

[2] See Ph. Van Haute & H. Westerink, 'Hysterie, Sexualität und Psychiatrie: Eine Relektüre der ersten Ausgabe der *Drei Abhandlungen zur Sexualtheorie*', in: S. Freud, *Drei Abhandlungen zur Sexualtheorie (1905)*, Chr. Huber, Ph. Van Haute & H. Westerink (Eds.). Vienna University Press, Vienna, 2015, 9-56.
[3] See Freud's footnote added in 1923 ('Fragment', p. 117).
[4] See J. Allouch, 'Freud embringue dans l'homosexualité feminine', in: *Cliniques mediteranéennes* 65 (2002), pp. 105-130; J. Allouch, *Ombre de ton chien: discours psychanalytique, discours lesbian*. Paris: Epel 2004; P. Gherovici, *Please Select Your Gender. From the Invention of Hysteria to the Democratizing of Transgenderism*. New York: Routledge, 2010.
[5] Freud, 'Fragment', p. 48.
[6] Ibid.
[7] Ibid., p. 13.

each one of Dora's bodily symptoms.[8] He takes on the position of an attorney who cross-examines a witness rather than a psychoanalyst who treats a patient when he insists that Dora was only seeking revenge against Mr K. Freud falls into the role of 'the one who knows' and the one who uses his subject, in this case Dora, to benefit his own cause and to serve his own theoretical ambitions.

> "When I informed her of this conclusion [that she was in love with Mr K., JWB] she did not assent to it. It is true that she at once told me that other people besides (one of her cousins, for instance – a girl who had stopped with them for some time at B—) had said to her: 'Why you're simply wild about that man!' But she herself could not be got to recollect any feelings of the kind."[9]

Freud's friendly bias towards Mr K. also reveals itself in the small side comment, again reserved in a footnote, when he wonders why Dora's reaction to Mr K. was so strong:

> "The question then arises: If Dora loved Herr K., what was the reason for her refusing him in the scene by the lake? Or at any rate, why did her refusal take such a brutal form, as though she was embittered against him? And how could a girl who was in love feel insulted by a proposal which was made in a manner neither tactless nor offensive?"[10]

With his ardent wish to prove Dora right, Freud is seized into the structure of Dora's life who had been a servant to the most intimate people in her life and constituted a pivotal object of their exchanges. Dora was beset by a torrent of unstable and contradictory identifications which in turn were characterized by displacements and condensations of both pre-Oedipal and Oedipal elements. Akin to the structure of a symbolic chain which Lacan elaborates in *The Purloined Letter* (1970) Dora's story follows a similar pattern of triangulated patterns, where each figure takes up a different position of knowledge and power at any one point in these interlocking structures. Dora circulates like a pirouette in a mix of erotic triangles

---

[8] See Freud's remark in a footnote: "The causes of Dora's disgust at the kiss were certainly not adventious, for in that case she could not have failed to remember and mention them. I happen to know Mr K., for he was the same person who had visited me with the patient's father (p.19), and he was still quite young and of prepossessing appearance". Freud, 'Fragment', p. 29.
[9] Ibid., p. 37.
[10] Ibid., p. 38.

1) between her parents, Philip and Käthe Bauer
2) between the K's, Hans K and Mrs K. (Peppina Zellenka)
3) between her father, Philip Bauer and Mrs K. (Peppina Zellenka)
4) between her father, Philip Bauer and the governess
5) between Mr K. (Herr Zellenka) and the governess
6) and possibly between Mr K. (Herr Zellenka) and Sigmund Freud.

Knowledge, secrets and omissions occupy a lot of space in this case, with Dora being the holder, keeper and 'revealer' of secrets. Her body functions as a fragment upon whom all the usual suspects inscribe their hidden desires and wished-for longings. Each one the figures, described above, make use of Dora for their own divided purposes, and in so doing, are rendering her mute.

Much like Anna O. Dora had found herself in the role of taking care of her sick father from an early age on. When Dora was six years old, her father had fallen ill of tuberculosis and the family had moved to Meran where it was primarily Dora who was nursing him back to health. Again, much like Anna O. and later Anna Freud, Dora continued to be in the role of the primary care-taker of her father, replacing thereby her mother in this pivotal Oedipal position. Even though, Dora most likely knew about the affair between her father and Mrs K. and made herself an accomplice in this affair to sustain her father and to act out her Oedipal resentment towards her mother, she nonetheless resented being handed over to Mr K., so that the father could continue his affair with Mrs K. Alternatively, Dora was also rendered speechless by Mrs K's use of her as a baby-sitter of the Ks' children as this task again strengthened Dora's premature Oedipal wish to be in the role of the powerful care-taker and also constituted a fulfillment of her unconscious, homosexual wish to be in close physical contact with Mrs K. And yet, it is at the same time very likely that Mrs K. used this as a ruse to distract Dora from her affair with Dora's father.

Dora thus swirls from one intimate space into another, touching upon the father's, Mrs K's and the mother's interior spaces, finding herself in the midst of all these spaces, eventually without a key. The latter was probably provided by Mr K. himself. Spyros Papapetros writes:

"This and other adjancencies as well as displacements and substitutions between movements, fluids, sounds, and spaces demonstrate that the walls of buildings and other architectural partitions in dream descriptions act mainly as permeable thresholds, alternatively facilitating and/or blocking movement. What we experience is not only 'substitution' and 'displacement', but also a form of transference, where feelings, qualities and attachments are sympathetically transported less between human subjects but rather between the spaces these subjects are inhabiting and dreaming. Such transferences appear to occur among the various individual rooms, and within the clustering of these spaces, as in the sequence of enfiladed rooms in Dora's childhood house in Vienna and later the hotel her family and the K.s temporarily occupied."[11]

I think Papapetros is right to emphasize the close proximity of rooms and spaces in Dora's life where all the central figures are living so closely with one another and enter so eagerly and one might even say, noisily, into Dora's life. Everyone, including the governess, knows of Mr Bauer's syphilis which he handed over to his wife. Most adult figures probably knew of Mr Bauer's affair with Mrs Zellenka (Mrs K), witnessing with greater or less intense scrutiny how the youngest female of them all moved in between these figures and spaces, finding only her desk as the one closed space in which she can keep her inner-most thoughts and worries. Only Mrs Bauer, Dora's mother, keeps to herself, not joining the whole circle of intrigues, encapsulating herself in a daily routine of cleaning up the whole mess around her.

Emma and Dora, the forgotten trauma theory, a case of Nachträglichkeit?

Before I address the prominent Freudian oversights of the transference relationship and Dora's homosexual love towards Mrs K, both tucked away in later-added footnotes in 1923, I would like to draw attention to another oversight which filters through this case. It is likely that Freud had forgotten or needed to disavow his earlier theory of trauma when he completed Dora's case history. In 'The Project' (1895) Freud narrates the story of a young girl Emma whose symptoms consist of not being able to go shopping on her own when she reaches adolescence. Whenever she enters into a store, she is overcome by fright and is compelled to leave the store. Freud discovers through Emma's narrations that her fright and ensuing phobic actions were based upon *two scenes*, one laying upon the other in separate intervals of time. He explains in 'The Project' that Emma had gone to a grocery store when she was eight years old to buy sweets. The shopkeeper had grabbed her genitals through her clothes and had laughed when he touched her. In spite of this first scene, Emma had nonetheless gone back a few more times to buy sweets again but then had stopped altogether

---

[11] S. Papapetros, 'Drop Form: Freud, Dora, and Dream Space', in: A. Sarnitz & I. Scholz-Strasser (Eds.), *Private Utopia. Cultural Setting of the Interior in the 19th and 20th Century*. Berlin/Boston: De Gruyter, 2015, pp. 58-88, p. 65.

going when she was eight years old. Years later however, when Emma reaches the age of fourteen, she goes back to another store where different store keepers are laughing (for an entirely different reason) when she enters the store. It is at this moment that Emma becomes frightened and has to leave the store. This second scene awakens the memory of the first scene and is now connected with the sensation of a sexual release with which she immediately re-invests *retroactively* the first scene, which in turn leaves her at age fourteen with a great sense of fright and shame. Freud comments:

> "Here we have the case of a memory arousing an affect which it did not arouse as an experience, because in the meantime the change [brought about] in puberty had made possible a different understanding of what was remembered.
> Now this case is typical of repression in hysteria. We invariably find that a memory is repressed which has only become a trauma by *deferred action*. The cause of this state of things is the retardation of puberty as compared with the rest of the individual's development."[12]

Freud's insight into the dynamics of *Nachträglichkeit* radically reshapes his theory about trauma and psychic functioning altogether. It leads him, I think, to reclaim his theory of neuroses where he had famously declared to Wilhelm Fliess in 1897 that "I no longer believe in *my neurotica*".[13] Through *Nachträglichkeit* Freud realizes that an external event in and of itself does not have enough weight to evoke a traumatic/symptomatic effect. The sheer memory of an event, saturated with the wished-for emotion or a wished-for fantasy could produce a similar devastating outcome. For an experience to have a traumatic effect, it had to re-occur at least one more time in two separate scenes, to produce its traumatic effects. Bernard Toboul analyzes Freud's early model of trauma with the following observation:

> "A temporality in two moments characterizes trauma, in terms of psychoanalysis, and distinguishes itself from the common model of shock. It defines itself by what happens afterwards where the efficiency of the second moment brings out and makes come into being what has been but could not be said, that is to say what was not. So the experience emerges, according to what was impossible, unspeakable so to say, impossible to

---

[12] S. Freud, 'Project For A Scientific Psychology' (1895), *SE* 1, p. 356.
[13] *The Complete Letters of Sigmund Freud to Wilhelm Fliess 1887–1904*, J.M. Masson (Ed.). Cambridge, MA: The Belknap Press of Harvard University Press 1985, p. 264.

bear, originally repressed and erased, and this unspeakable charges itself with a sexual meaning that remains estranged to some extent. Trauma allows us to symbolize through après-coup yet it maintains a zone of inaccessibility. It is this inaccessibility that returns in repetition."[14]

Toboul remarks that Freud's early theory of trauma cannot be fully understood if one does not know / sense the difference between *Erfahrung* ('experience') and *Erlebnis* ('lived event'). Whereas English has only one word for both, the German language has two distinct words for something that was only lived, maybe simply noted *(Erlebnis)* as Freud describes in the first scene, while experience *(Erfahrung)*, as it occurs in the second scene, is a lived through experience within which Emma can more fully symbolize what had not been possible to fully live through when she was a young girl.[15]

A similar sequence of two scenes, one layering upon one another, occurs in the case of Dora when Freud describes Dora's first erotic encounter in the store with Mr K. after they had watched the church parade. In that moment of writing, it appears as if Freud had forgotten his own notion of *Nachträglichkeit* (afterwardsness / deferred action) when he describes Dora's disgust at Mr K. "pressing a kiss on her lip"[16] (p.28). Instead of viewing this as the first scene of an encounter that will unfold to be a traumatic one later on when Mr K. kisses her again at the lake, Freud insists that Dora should have reacted with excitement rather than mere disgust. It is puzzling why he does not link up at any moment the scene at the church parade with Dora's later visit at the church in Dresden where she longingly contemplates the image of the Madonna. Freud mentions the various suicide threats and deaths in Dora's life, the father's thought of suicide, the aunt's death, Dora's own suicide letter hidden in her desk and the near suicide of Mr K. when she encounters him again in the streets after they had broken off the relationship, as he is run over by a carriage, staring at her. Yet Freud never connects these losses, near and potential losses with one another in a meaningful way, leaving Dora speechless once again, as she witnesses the near death of Mr K. Since her prominent symptom of aphonia

---

[14] B. Toboul, 'Remarques introductives a la question du trauma', in: *Figures de la psychanalyse* 8 (2003/1), app. 1-3, p. 1. Translation JWB.

[15] See D.W. Winnicott, 'Fear of breakdown' (1971/1974), in: D.C. Winnicott, R. Shepherd & M. Davis (Eds.), *Psychoanalytic Explorations*. Cambridge, MA: Harvard University Press, 1989, pp. 87-95, and Thomas Odgen's discussion of Winnicott's paper for a different, yet closely akin theory of Freud's early theory of trauma: 'Fear of breakdown and the unlived life', in: *Reclaiming unlived life. Experiences in Psychoanalysis*. New York: Routledge, 2016, pp. 47-70.

[16] Freud, 'Fragment', p. 28.

appears at that moment, what is it that prevents Freud to ask himself retroactively (*nachträglich*) what other painful losses Dora might have endured and witnessed that had rendered her so voiceless in her early adolescence. Freud's theoretical zeal to prove that sexuality was the key to explain hysterical symptoms and the problem of psycho-neuroses, renders him blind, I think, to his earlier theory of trauma which had not emphasized sexuality in a similarly strong manner, but had privileged the back and forth movement of *Nachträglichkeit* as an internal psychic process that re-invests an earlier (possibly unlived, unsymbolized) experience with a newly discovered sexual sensation.

Dora and the homosexual woman – Ida Bauer versus Margarethe von Trauttenegg

Let me turn now to the question of hysteria and perversion and see where the difference between those two structures lies. I have wondered whether Dora, after all these years, could now be seen as a woman situated in a perverse structure, or whether she remains the hysteric heroine whom we have come to know her by now. My hypothesis is that Dora survived a perverse household through her hysterical structure, by submitting to remain an object of trade which had first been sacrificed by her mother, then by her father, and subsequently by Mr K. and Mrs K., for whom and through whom she finally becomes a subject, first speaking through her symptoms, but eventually also speaking in her own name. Hysterics are considered the truest historians because they will not cease to speak the truth of the unconscious, and in that sense, Dora has become a monument (*Denk- und Mahnmal*) of the hysteric, searching for and speaking the truth. A comparison with the case of the homosexual woman, makes clear that a different structure is at work in Dora's case than in the homosexual woman's case, despite the many similarities existing between them. Both women were young, intelligent and determined people, of Jewish, bourgeois descent, and both were brought to Freud with the plea "Please try and bring her to reason."[17] Both were afflicted by suicidal ideas, with Dora expressing them in a letter she hides, and with the homosexual woman actually making a suicide attempt at the Kettenbrückengasse railway overpass, after she encountered her father as she was holding hands with 'la cocotte'. Their desperate suicidal attempts, one imagined and one enacted admonished their fathers to bring them to Professor Freud at Berggasse 19, and 'to bring them to reason'.

Jacques Lacan comments that these two cases perfectly complement themselves because both in their respective neurotic and perverse structures mix up the imaginary with the symbolic position, thereby illustrating Freud's well

---

[17] Ibid., p. 26.

known dictum that "perversion is the negative of neurosis".[18] Gherovici[19] and Allouch[20] also suggest through their readings of Lacan's texts that Freud went back to the case of Dora after he had completed the analysis of the homosexual woman (Margarethe von Trautenegg), realizing only through her analysis the importance of the homosexual nature of the hysteric's love object. In his seminar IV on *The Object Relation* (1956/1957), Lacan writes,

> "the hysteric is someone who loves vicariously, and you find in many case histories, that the hysteric is someone, whose object is homosexual – the hysteric approaches the homosexual object through the identification with someone of the other sex. (…) In other words, through Mr K., in as much as she is Mr K., at the imaginary point which represents the personality of Mr K., this is where Dora is attached to the figure of Mrs K."[21]

What are the differences between the two cases and why are they so interconnected and enlightening of one another?

In the case of Dora, the mother is relegated to the background, and even though, she is being described as unintelligent and suffering from a "cleaning psychosis", Dora is strongly identified with her through her various symptoms, primarily in the end, the symptom from which she would eventually die, i.e. stomach cancer. In the case of the homosexual woman, the mother is present, stealing away from her daughter, the attention her husband is lavishing upon her. In other words, she robs her daughter of the father's attention and pays little, if at all, jealous attention to her. In the case of Dora, it is the father who introduces 'a third woman, Mrs K' into the triangle, in the case of the homosexual woman, it is the patient herself, who introduces the 'third woman', 'the cocotte', into the triangle.

Freud discovers relatively quickly in Dora's case that she is the hidden pivotal support of the illicit relationship/affair between her father and Mrs K. She benefits from that knowledge, it makes her stand in the position of the imaginary phallus who believes that she is in the possession of the entire truth. Indeed, everyone comes to her to tell her their side of their story, including the governesses and the aunts. This illicit and powerful knowledge also gives her

---

[18] See, J. Lacan, J. *Le Seminaire IV. La relation d'objet*. Paris: Edition du Seuil, 1994, p. 136.
[19] See, Gherovici, *Please select your gender.*
[20] See, Allouch, 'Freud embringue dans l'homosexualité feminine'; Allouch, *Ombre de ton chien.*
[21] J. Lacan, *Le séminare IV. La relation d'objet*. Paris: Editions du Seuil, 1994, p. 138. Translation JWB.

the opportunity to be close to Mrs K, identifying with her position and even becoming the maternal substitute for her children. Knowing and keeping silent about the affair allows her close bodily contact with Mrs K's (Peppina's) white marbled body and permits her an intimate introduction into sexual matters via the lecture of Mantegazza. Lacan writes in *Seminar VIII*:

> "Dora would not be a hysteric, if she was satisfied with her phantasm. She aims at something else, something better, she looks for the Great Other. She aims at the great Other. I have explained for some time that Mrs K. is for her the incarnation of the question, *What is a woman?* That is why on the level of the fantasm, the *fading* of the subject to the little *a* does not come about, but something else happens."[22]

Dora, unlike a paranoid subject believes in the great Other, even though the father is impotent, but precisely because the father is impotent, is lacking, Dora, in true hysteric fashion makes it her business to support the father, the idealized, castrated father through her support of his affair with Mrs K. Lacan calls Dora "la procureuse de ce signe": the procurator of the sign within an imaginary form. Dora, like most hysterics, does everything to fill up the Other.

> "The devotion of the hysteric, her passion to identify herself with all the sentimental dramas, to be there, to support everything which plays behind the backdrops with so much passion even though it is not her business, it is there that she is driven, it is the source from which all her behavior and actions emerge. She sacrifices her desire for this sign. She prefers something other than her desire, she prefers that her desire remain unsatisfied, that the Other keep the keys to her mystery."[23]

Dora desires as though she is Mr K., constructing her desire in the place of the Other. She loves Mrs K. from the position of her identification with Mr K. In contrast to the homosexual woman, Dora has a father, who is lacking, who is impotent, and it is that paternal lack which causes and maintains Dora's desire. Dora remains so attached to the father because he is lacking and she desires something beyond him, namely the one he desires, Mrs K. Dora loves her father for what he does not give, so that she can maintain the illusion of filling him up, of sustaining him. The structure falls apart when Herr K. utters the words,

---

[22] J. Lacan, *Le Seminaire VIII. Le Transfer*. Paris: Editions du Seuil, 1991, p. 293. Translation JWB.
[23] Ibid., p. 293-294. Translation JWB.

"Ich habe nichts von meiner Frau": "(…) I get nothing out of my wife."[24]. In that moment the triadic structure crumbles because Mrs K. is enthroned through the words of Mr K. and suddenly Mr K. is only available for Dora without the mediation through Mrs K. It is at this point that she slaps Mr K. in the face at the Garda Lake. Dora sees herself suddenly only as the object of Mr K.'s desire and cannot bear being only the object of a man's desire. Lacan summarizes the case in his book on *Psychoses* (1981). He writes:

> "Who is Dora? She is someone trapped in a very clear symptomatic state, with the qualifications that Freud, by his own admission, makes a mistake over the object of Dora's desire in that he himself is too centered the question of the object, that is, in that he doesn't bring out the fundamental subjective duality implicated in it. He asks himself what Dora desires, before asking himself who desires in Dora. And in the end, Freud realizes that in this quartet – Dora, her father, Herr und Frau K. – Frau K. is the object that really interests Dora, in so far as she is identified with Herr K. The question of where Dora's ego is located is thus resolved – Herr K. is Dora's ego."[25]

The homosexual woman, in contrast, has a father who is not lacking, who is promising her unconsciously a baby of his own. It is as if the homosexual patient is attempting to show her father what true love is by presenting him with a woman who does not have what he has, but who can be what he has, i.e. the phallus. So the homosexual woman constructs herself a situation of possible lack to keep her desire moving, but she is only displacing the function from one place to the other and is thereby enacting her desire right in front of the father's eyes. The homosexual woman is not a procurator of signs but a procurator of acts and when these acts fail, she is confronted with a void, which compels her to this desperate act of attempting to kill herself. In the case history of the homosexual woman, everything is open, visible and to be seen, whereas, in Dora's case, everything is veiled, hidden and concealed.

In the end, when the homosexual woman's desired scene succeeds and she is seen by her father with the scandalous *cocotte*, the imagined scene goes awry with her father becoming furious at this sight and the cocotte becoming enraged at the homosexual woman's fragile desire, telling her to get lost. In that moment, the

---

[24] Ibid., p. 98.
[25] J. Lacan, *The Psychoses. The Seminar of Jacques Lacan: Book III 1955-1956*, J.-A. Miller (Ed.), New York: Taylor and Francis, 1993, p. 174ff.

homosexual woman is without any means to keep the illusion alive of having found the paternal phallus in the cocotte. Abandoned by both, in a *passage à l'acte,* she throws herself over the fence onto the train station. In this suicidal act, as she throws herself down onto the train tracks, the homosexual woman realizes her unconscious wish to have a baby from her father. Freud unveils this wish through the word play of '*niederkommen*' which means both 'to come down' and 'to give birth' in German.

In the end, it becomes possible to see how Dora realizes similar phantasies and wishes but lives them through her symptoms and hidden identifications, whereas the homosexual woman (Margarethe von Trautenegg) enacts them, displays them, and only finds refuge in acting them out under the eyes of others. Thus we can realize how these two women, forever intimately linked in Freud's mind, come to represent one of the major differences existing between neurosis and perversion, with the neurotic repressing the perverse pleasures that the perverse subject openly displays.

In conclusion

Freud's failed case of Dora remains a story that leaves many traces behind, some of which have and can only be uncovered in a movement of *Nachträglichkeit*. It took a great deal of courage for Freud to publish this case in the first place, even though he presents himself as a self-assured conquistador, yet narrates a case in which he was fired and in which he presented his clinical work in a rather unfavorable light. Never before or after, did he show himself to be so directive and over-bearing to a young patient, not interpreting her symptoms, but nearly inter-penetrating them. And yet it is precisely Freud's willingness to publish this failure and to publish it with a four-year delay, only to return to it twenty years later which makes it such an instructive, lively and enigmatic one. So many possibilities and interpretive perspectives open up in hind-sight, engaging the reader in a constant play of foreshadowing and backshadowing between the present and past of the case, but also the future from which the case is being consistently explored again, that Dora remains the *roman à clef* that Freud intended her to be from the very beginning.

On the Signification of Dora's Father

Ulrike Kadi

Since Freud has written about Dora's treatment, her case has been taken up for discussion from different angles, including her neurotic symptoms,[1] her traumatic experiences,[2] her adolescence,[3] her gender,[4] her homosexual desire,[5] her later life,[6] Freud's choice of her pseudonym,[7] his handling of (counter-) transference,[8] the new genre of text[9] Freud was inventing with this piece of writing about a patient and much more.[10] In this paper, we intend to look at a less frequently considered crucial point of her story: her father. His outstanding contribution to her development and to several possibly traumatic experiences she had is, of course, beyond question. Here his role will be discussed with a focus on both Freud's view on him and Lacan's comments on Freud's text.

---

[1] P. Marty, M. Fain, M. de M'Uzan & C. David, 'Le cas Dora et le point de vue psychosomatique', in: *Revue Française de Psychanalyse* XXXII (1968), pp. 679-714.
[2] R.B. Blass, 'Did Dora have an Oedipus Complex – A Reexamination of the Theoretical Context of Freud's "Fragment of an Analysis"', in: *Psychoanalytic Study of the Child* 47 (1992), pp. 159-187.
[3] V. King, *Die Urszene der Psychoanalyse. Adoleszenz und Geschlechterspannung im Fall Dora*. Stuttgart: Verlag Internationale Psychoanalyse, 1995.
[4] H. Cixous, *Le portrait de Dora*. Paris: des femmes, 1986.
[5] J. Moscovitz, 'D'un signe qui lui serait fait ou aspects de l'homo-sexualité dans "Dora"', in: *Revue Française de Psychanalyse* XXXVII (1973), pp. 359-372; A. Ruhs, 'Freud 1919: Ein Fall von weiblicher Homosexualität und gewisse Folgen', in: C. Diercks & S. Schlülter (Eds.), *Sigmund Freud Vorlesungen 2006. Die großen Krankengeschichten*. Vienna: Mandelbaum, 2008, pp. 135-144.
[6] F. Deutsch, 'A Footnote to Freud's "Fragment of an Analysis of a Case of Hysteria"', in: *Psychoanalytic Quarterly* 26 (1957), pp.159-167.
[7] H.S. Decker, 'The Choice of a Name: "Dora" and Freud's Relationship with Breuer', in: *Journal of the American Psychoanalytic Association* 30 (1982), pp. 113-136. See also, J.-M. Rabaté, 'Dora's Gift; or, Lacan's Homage to Dora', in: *Psychoanalytic Inquiry* 25:1 (2005), p. 92.
[8] J. Lacan, 'Intervention sur le transfert', *Écrits*. Paris: Seuil, 1966, pp. 215-226. G.J. Makari, 'Dora's Hysteria and the Maturation of Sigmund Freud's Transference Theory: A New Historical Interpretation', in: *Journal of the American Psychoanalytic Association* 45 (1997), pp. 1061-1096. J. Glenn, 'Freud, Dora, and the Maid: A Study of Countertransference', in: *Journal of the American Psychoanalytic Association* 34 (1986), pp. 591-606.
[9] S. Marcus, 'Freud and Dora. Story, History, Case History', in: C. Bernheimer & C. Kahane (Eds.), *In Dora's Case. Freud – Hysteria – Feminism*. New York: Columbia University Press, 1985, pp. 56-91.
[10] All of these works are just a few examples out of the vast number of references to Dora's case. For an early attempt to standardize these references, see Bernheimer & Kahane, *In Dora's Case*. For a later attempt, see King, *Urszene*.

This twofold glimpse allows us to examine in detail particular aspects of how the approach to the father's role evolved within psychoanalysis over the last century. It is chosen to provide a thick description of this approach from the perspective of two authors – Freud and Lacan – during a time characterized by a far-reaching cultural shift in the social role of the father.

I

Dora's (= Ida Bauer's) father, Philipp, was a migrant within the Austrian multi-ethnic state[11] who came from a poor background in Bohemia close to Iglau (Jíhlava). He had a sister, who was a little older than him, and an older brother. Philipp moved to Vienna shortly after marrying Katharina Gerber. They first lived in a flat at Berggasse 32 and later settled in Liechtensteinstraße. Both places were not far from Freud's flat in Berggasse. As a textile manufacturer, Dora's father was a hardworking, wealthy man who owned two factories, one in Nachòd and the other close to the Saxonian border in Warnsdorf (Varnsdorf). He demanded as much from the workers in his factories as from himself. Philipp had classical liberal views, advocating freedom of speech and press, disestablishment and universal suffrage excluding women and lower class people. With his thinking and his way of life, he represented the modern type of a middle-class bourgeois in Vienna around 1900. Personally he was described as a bright and charming man. Bauer was a Freemason, and he was in charge of charity work at his lodge.

Philipp was also not a healthy man. He was the first of the Bauer family whom Freud got to know because he asked Freud for help long before Dora's analysis.[12] In 1892, when Dora was ten years old, her father suffered from several somatic symptoms (like retinal detachment and impaired vision), followed two years later by a bout of confusion accompanied by signs of paralysis and unspecified psychic disorders. Freud suspected a syphilitic infection, which turned out to be the right guess, because the symptoms vanished after antiluetic treatment.[13] Another disease also had a great impact on the Bauers' life: aged six, Dora had to move to Meran with her family because of her father's tuberculosis, which necessitated relocation to a southern and warmer climate.

On the other hand, his poor state of health was no big deal, as Dora and her father were surrounded by loved ones suffering from a number of medical

---

[11] For the biographical data mentioned below, see W. Maderthaner, 'Von der Zeit um 1860 zum Jahr 1945', in: *Wien. Geschichte einer Stadt*. Band 3, P. Csendes & F. Oppl (Eds.), Vienna: Böhlau, 2006, p. 275ff.

[12] S. Freud, 'Fragment of an Analysis of a Case of Hysteria (1905 [1901])', *SE* 7, p. 19.

[13] Ibid., p. 19.

conditions. Philipp's two elder siblings are mentioned as being in poor health, too: His unhappy sister, whom Freud diagnosed as suffering from psychoneurosis, died from a sudden wasting disease, even though the precise cause of death was never determined. Philipp's single brother was called a "hypochondriac bachelor"[14] by Freud, which does not sound healthy either.[15] And last, but not least, Freud inferred that Philipp's wife suffered from a special form of psychic disturbance, which he gave the ironic name of "housewife's psychosis"[16].

It almost goes without saying that Dora's father determined much more than the family's place of living. In Freud's case history, Philipp becomes the pivot of Dora's story in many respects. It is he who introduces his daughter to Freud. It is his relationship with Freud that allows him to provide anamnestic details about the patient. This is not without difficulty, as Philipp is part of his daughter's life reality and of the stories she tells to her analyst. More than that, he is a key player in the story involving the K. family, which has intense effects on Dora's state. He is a central object in Dora's phantasies and dreams. And above all, he shapes the transference in Dora's relation to her analyst.

Philipp did not take his daughter to Freud after Dora had written a suicide letter which he and his wife found. While he was shocked by her action, which he considered above all an attempt to frighten her parents, it was not until her first hysteric attack when she fainted that he insisted on her seeing Freud. Freud emphasized that it was her father who referred Dora to psychoanalysis, and there is no indication that Freud ever asked her whether she herself was interested in a talking cure.[17]

II

Freud listened to Philipp's version of Dora's story while keeping in mind that he had to hear other people's versions of what was going on before reasoning about the case.[18] Freud's attitude towards Dora's father was benevolent and friendly before Dora's treatment started. He praises Philipp as an intelligent, gifted[19] and insightful man because he was not overwhelmed by Dora's suicidal innuendos.[20] Freud appears to be even more sympathetic to the father when

---

[14] Ibid., p. 19.
[15] Dora's own symptoms, too, are treated as difficulties resulting from medical problems: In Freud's interpretation of the first dream, her bed-wetting as a child and her masturbation are perceived to be of clinical value. See ibid., p. 74.
[16] Ibid., p. 20.
[17] Ibid., p. 23. King assumes that Dora actually wished to change. King, *Urszene*, p. 100.
[18] Freud, 'Fragment', p. 26.
[19] Ibid., p. 18.
[20] Ibid., p. 23.

we compare his remarks about Philipp with those about Käthe Bauer, Dora's mother. His approach to her figure remains reproachful and pale, which is in stark contrast to the role he theoretically ascribes to the mother figure and her outstanding contribution to the development of the child.[21]

But Freud's opinion of Philipp Bauer seems to change in the course of Dora's treatment. As soon as Dora enters his treatment room, it is no longer Philipp who is Freud's link to Dora; instead, Dora's view of her father shapes Freud's thoughts about him.[22] In this shift, the extraordinary manufacturer becomes a weak man. Freud at last starts to agree with Dora's accusation that the father is using her as an object of barter[23] to hide his own love affair. Freud notices Philipp's sexual impotence.[24] And in the end, he realizes that he will disappoint Philipp's expectations. Freud then calls him "never entirely straightforward",[25] remarking that he had no ambitions to hide the father's liaison with Mrs K. from the daughter or anyone else.

From Freud's psychoanalytic perspective, Philipp's role in Dora's unconscious is shaped by two elements: her sexual feelings towards her father (and his successors like Mr K.) and her identification with him and his objects, Mrs K. and her mother. Freud's interpretations of her dreams serve to justify this view on her sexual feelings. Mr K.'s sexual advances towards Dora that lead to her first dream are taken as part of an infantile wishful complex to be her father's beloved partner. Dora wishes to be tempted by her father.[26]

Freud's way of discussing this topic in her case marks a shift in his theoretical presuppositions: Until the late 1890s, he worked with the seduction hypothesis when confronted with stories of hysteric patients about sexual abuse. As long as Freud took his patients' stories as historical truth, he and his readers were faced with the fact that many of his patients' relatives and acquaintances were to blame for sexual abuse. Already some years before Freud started working on Dora's case, he found another way of thinking about the stories his patients told him. Without calling into question the traumatic impact of experiences on

---

[21] See I. Erlich, 'What Happened to Jocasta?', in: *Bulletin of the Menninger Clinic* 41 (1977), pp. 280-284. On the same topic, see also E. H. Spitz, 'Freud's Women', in: *Psychoanalytic Quarterly* 64 (1995), pp. 177-180, p. 179; K. K. Lewin, 'Dora Revisited', in: *Psychoanalytic Review* 60 (1973-74), pp. 519-532; T. Moi, 'Representation of Patriarchy. Sexuality and Epistemology in Freud's Dora', in: *In Dora's Case*, pp. 181-199.

[22] King points to a certain reluctance on the part of Freud to change his mind about Philipp Bauer (King, Urszene, p. 16).

[23] S. Freud, 'Fragment, p. 34.

[24] Ibid., p. 47.

[25] Ibid., p. 109.

[26] Ibid., p. 87.

the patients and thereby accepting their genetic truth,[27] he traced their content back to phantasies, known as Oedipal phantasies, which regularly occur during childhood.[28] The father is no longer seen as an external agent primarily based on his role in reality, but mainly as the fantasized object of the little girl's sexual wishes. This shift has far-reaching consequences: The father is no longer to blame for his daughter's neurosis – it is she who is made responsible for her symptoms, in Dora's case especially when Freud links them to her masturbatory activities during childhood.[29]

Dora's father nevertheless remains a central focus of Freud's treatment because he is part of her psychic life. He serves as a protagonist in both dreams Freud analyzes during the cure. In the first dream, the father says he is concerned about his two children getting burnt, while in the second he is mentioned as a dead man who was in ill health before. In her first dream, the father serves as a haven for Dora, who is overwhelmed by feelings of disgust following the kiss incident with Mr K.; in the second dream, Dora describes a situation in which she has left her father, which Freud at the end of his text takes as a prediction of her later marriage.[30] In her dreams, Dora returns to her father and then leaves him. This movement repeats itself in her treatment: Dora approaches Freud and eventually leaves him, too. But Freud seems to be very cautious to acknowledge that he functioned as a father in Dora's transference.

In the eleven-week period between entering and leaving psychoanalysis, the shadows of Dora's sexually connoted relationship with her father and his followers in transference are not the only experiences she talks about. During her talking cure she reveals her father to be her primary object of identification.[31] Freud does not pay too much attention to this – maybe because there are also moments of (developmentally speaking) earlier identifications with a potentially dangerous impact on Freud which in transference might have involved him: With Philipp, Dora shares symptoms of ill health. Besides the phantasy of oral sex being expressed by a "tickling in her throat",[32] her coughing can be understood

---

[27] For the difference between historic and genetic truth, see E. Erikson, 'Reality and Actuality. An Address', in: *In Dora's Case*, pp. 44-55.
[28] Freud, 'Fragment', p. 56ff. Blass finds four different formulations of the seduction hypothesis and shows that there are fragments of it left in Freud's handling of the Dora case. R.B. Blass, 'Did Dora have an Oedipus Complex'.
[29] Freud, 'Fragment', p. 78. Concerning the historical and medical background of Freud's argumentation, see also C. Bonomi, 'The relevance of castration and circumcision to the origins of psychoanalysis: 1. The medical context', in: *The International Journal of Psychoanalysis* 90 (2009), pp. 551-580.
[30] Freud, 'Fragment', p. 122.
[31] See H.S. Decker, *Freud, Dora, and Vienna 1900*. New York: Free Press, 1991, p. 195.
[32] Freud, 'Fragment', p. 48.

as a form of identification with her father, which Freud regards as regressive.[33] Depending on the level of her regression, Dora reaches an Oedipal or even pre-Oedipal level in her phantasies.[34] In the latter case, instead of having a love relationship with her father, she, through her cough, imitates him like a child mimics her mother on a bodily level. The distinction between the father figure and the mother figure becomes blurred. Taking the symptom that way opens up its (oral) aggressive potential: Whoever is the focus of Dora's identification is under threat because he or she might be bitten or even swallowed.

The signification of Dora's father has multiple facets. Her case was an early one for Freud, who later discovered more details of the paternal functioning, thereby developing a richer picture of the father's signification.[35] In the Dora case, the following significations of the father in real life can be identified: In the beginning, Philipp stands for a potent man who is successful in his work. But he is also a sick man whose weakness is depicted by Freud when Dora's perspective of her father starts to prevail.[36] And his prowess is not only limited by his poor state of bodily health, but by the fact that he is a liar. The father tried to keep Dora in the dark about his relationship with Mrs K. and used the daughter like a shield to hide his affair from others. Dora knew about his ordinary love affair.[37] And she remained calm about it.

Dora had several reasons for keeping her father's secret. Freud's interpretations focused on the Oedipal relationship with her father and no longer on a scandal of incestuous seduction of the father, which had been the main thrust of his earlier approach to hysteric phenomena. He focused on the sexual wishes not of the father but of Dora *vis-à-vis* her father and his successors in transference. In addition to and interwoven with the Oedipal axis, Dora wishes to be like her father, whom she idealizes and identifies with – maybe on an early pre-Oedipal level. In any case, she is caught in a maze of hysteric wishes and beliefs concerning her father and his love affair.

There are facets of the father's role Freud seems to have been less interested in: One might speculate that Dora's father served as a protection against a discontented mother or similar uncomfortable concerns in her life. Freud asserts that Dora has a poor relationship with her mother and claims that she once

---

[33] S. Freud, 'Group Psychology and the Analysis of the Ego (1921)', *SE 18*, p. 107.
[34] For a pre-Oedipal interpretation of the act of reading in Dora's case, see S. Van Den Berg, 'Reading and Writing Dora: Pre-Oedipal Conflict in Freud's "Fragment of an Analysis of a Case of Hysteria"', in: *Psychoanalysis and Contemporary Thought* 10 (1987/1), pp. 45-67.
[35] See, P. Bruno, *Le père et ses noms*. Paris: Érès, 2000, pp. 9-66.
[36] Bruno (ibid., p.14) stresses Freud's ambivalence towards the father in the Dora case. To my mind, Freud's view on Philipp Bauer clearly changed when Freud accepted Dora's approach.
[37] Freud, 'Fragment', p. 31.

became obnoxious in her analysis while identifying with her mother.[38] Freud only regrets not having followed the track of the father's statement in Dora's first dream that he does not want his children to perish.[39] One might speculate whether Freud was reluctant to clearly realize Dora's wish to be protected by her father, which in transference could be understood as what Dora wished for from Freud.

Another feature of the father and his psychic impact remains rather neglected at this early stage of Freud's theories: the father's death in Dora's second dream, which Freud mainly interprets as revenge. He has not yet discovered the symbolic function of the father, which is closely linked to the absence of the father and his death. In Dora's case, Freud perceives the power of transference in its far-reaching scope. He seems overwhelmed by it, at certain points hesitating in his interpretations of Dora's affectionate state towards his own person.[40] The fire of transference and the concomitant disappointment when Dora leaves him might be one reason why Freud's view of his patient stuck to a heterosexual matrix and why he failed to realize the lesbian facets of Dora's phantasy for so long.

III

Lacan's contributions to the signification of Dora's father were made almost half a century after her treatment. Like Freud never saw President Schreber, Lacan never met Dora and her father. His comments on her analysis are purely text-based using Freud's description of the case. Lacan further elaborated his theories about the father and his function over the years,[41] and they go far beyond the comments he made on Freud's 'Fragment'. Here they can only be pointed to insofar as they are of interest to Lacan's reading of Dora.

Lacan already talked about Dora's case before developing his famous Name-of-the-Father concept. In 1951, in his small intervention on transference, Lacan introduces Dora's father as someone who shuts his eyes to a detestable encounter his daughter had to go through.[42] Lacan involves Freud in the case history by pointing to the fact that Philipp Bauer in fact lied to Freud after having confided in him earlier.[43] Here, Lacan diverges from Freud's view with

---

[38] Ibid., p. 20 and 74.
[39] Ibid., p. 91.
[40] See also King, *Urszene*, p. 93 ff.
[41] See also P. Bruno, *Le père et ses noms* and E. Porge, *Les noms du père chez Jacques Lacan. Ponctuations et problématiques*. Paris: Editions Érès, 1997.
[42] Lacan, 'Intervention', p. 218. For a critical feminist view on Lacan's remarks in this text, see S. Gearhart, 'The Scene of Psychoanalysis. The Unanswered Question of Dora', in: *In Dora's Case*, pp. 105-127.
[43] Lacan 'Intervention', p. 219.

respect to Dora's identification with the male figures in her life (her father, Mr K., Freud himself). Although within an Oedipal frame, Lacan's understanding is linked in a different way to Dora's remembrance of having sucked her left thumb while tugging on her brother's ear with her right hand.[44] Whereas Freud's remarks center on Dora's self-gratification of sucking a penis-shaped part of her own body, Lacan seems to be more interested in the figure of the brother.[45] He takes the little scene involving the brother as formative with respect to Dora's imagination about the significance of woman and man. And he doubts that the father is by nature an element of the Oedipus complex; to him, the prevalence of the father in the Oedipus complex has mainly normative reasons.[46]

When Lacan elaborates his position a few years later, he gravitates towards Freud's Oedipal view of the story. To him, the daughter's identification with the father has now become a necessary Oedipal detour because of the phallus, which has no equivalent on the female side.[47] Dora's father cannot serve in the way fathers usually do because he – a sick, weak, broken man – lacks the (symbolic) phallus. For Lacan, her father's phallic failure becomes central to Dora's position.[48]

Love, as a form of giving something one does not have, circulates around nothing. In this respect, the father's missing phallus could be a perfect gift[49] in the exchange between Dora and her father if there were no other subjects involved. The way Dora stabilizes her psychic position when faced with the love affair between her father and Mrs K. is an answer to her question what it is that Mrs K. loves in her father.[50] The answer is easy: It is the phallus. For Dora, Mrs K. becomes an incarnation of the female function which locates the phallus to have as belonging to the man, her father.[51] Dora concludes by analogy that she can tolerate the exchange between Mrs K. and her father as long as she can deem herself to be an involved third party who is loved by her father like Mrs K. In the scene at the lake, when Mr K. tells Dora that he failed to get anything out of his wife, the balance is destroyed: If there was no phallic

---

[44] Ibid., pp. 219-221.
[45] O. Hewitson, 'The Dora Parallax', see http://www.lacanonline.com/index/2014/08/the-dora-parallax/ (accessed on 31-5-2017).
[46] Lacan, 'Intervention', p. 223. See also Porge, *Les noms du père*, p. 33.
[47] J. Lacan, *Le Séminaire. Livre III (1955-1956). Les Psychoses*. Paris: Éditions du Seuil, 1981, p. 208.
[48] J. Lacan, *Le Séminaire. Livre IV (1956-1957). La relation d'objet*. Paris: Éditions du Seuil, 1994, p. 139.
[49] Concerning Lacan's understanding of the gift in this context, see Rabaté, 'Dora's Gift', pp. 84-93.
[50] Lacan, *La relation d'objet*, p. 141.
[51] Ibid., p. 141.

transmission between Mr and Mrs K., there would be no such transmission between Dora and her father either.[52]

During the 1950s, Lacan uses his categories of the symbolic, the imaginary and the real to unfold three manifestations of the father: the imaginary,[53] the symbolic and the real father. The Name-of-the-Father, also referred to as metaphor of the father, characterizes the father's symbolic role.[54] It designates the absent father, the dead father of Freud's *Totem and Taboo,* who as a metaphor serves to stabilize the subjective structure. The Name-of-the-Father soon becomes a crucial element in Lacan's reasoning about psychosis. For a long time, Lacan assumes the absence of the Name-of-the-Father in a subject to be the main characteristic of the psychotic structure.[55]

Of course, Lacan does not diagnose a psychotic structure in Dora, he only observes a psychotic phenomenon in her case history at the moment when she accuses her father of having deliberately delivered her to prostitution to hide his love affair with Mrs K.[56] The paranoid state for Lacan fits with Dora's hysteric problem of finding any access to her own desire. With her male identification, Dora has disguised herself with insignia of the Other. And in the moment at the lake when Mr K. confesses that he "[got] nothing out of [his] wife"[57] she falls back to a demand for love from her father.[58] Some years later, Lacan will call Dora's slapping in Mr K.'s face a *passage à l'acte,*[59] which is a way of overcoming a psychotic state.

The father, and especially Dora's father, as a vivid and concrete person is not given much room in Lacan's seminars. This does not come as a surprise given that Lacan never met him. But there is another reason for the absence of the concrete father figure: In Lacan's evolving, rather abstract way of speaking, the different aspects of the paternal function are increasingly split up: the O, or big Other, which represents the necessary support missing in psychotic

---

[52] Ibid., p.143.
[53] The imaginary father is the good father, the idealized father, the father as a rival who the child is competing with. Ibid., p. 220.
[54] Ibid., p. 364.
[55] For an overview of Lacan's theory of psychosis, see G. Morel, *Ambiguïtés sexuelles. Sexuation et psychose*. Paris: Anthropos, 2000; C. Fellahian, *La psychose selon Lacan. Évolution d'un concept*. Paris: L'Harmattan, 2005; M. Recalcati, 'Madness and Structure in Jacques Lacan', in: *lacanian ink* 2008 (32), pp. 97-121, S. Vanheule, *The Subject of Psychosis: A Lacanian Perspective*. New York, Basingstoke: Palgrave Macmillan, 2011.
[56] Lacan, *Les Psychoses*, p. 106.
[57] Freud, 'Fragment', p. 98.
[58] J. Lacan, *Le Séminaire. Livre V (1957-1958). Les formations de l'inconscient*. Paris: Éditions du Seuil, 1998, p. 370.
[59] J. Lacan, *Le Séminaire. Livre X (1962-1963). L'angoisse*. Paris: Éditions du Seuil, 2004, p. 137.

structures, the phallus, the Name-of-the-Father and the object a, little a, which as a phantasy can also carry paternal features. In Lacan's reading[60] of Dora's case, the question of how she manages her desire moves center stage. Mr K. gains in importance – he becomes object a. But the phantasy of Mr K.'s love is not Dora's main goal. She aims for the big O, which Lacan now detaches from the father. Instead, Mrs K., the adored woman, comes to occupy the position of O. Dora tries to represent an imaginary phallus that makes her impotent father potent, thereby stabilizing the relationship between Mrs K. and her father. Her desire is to support the father's desire.[61] She tries to complete the incomplete O because, as a hysteric, she cannot stand the castration (taken as an acceptance of lack in a general sense) of the big O.

The way Lacan approaches Dora's father develops over the years in parallel to his changing views on the hysteric structure.[62] Moments of a battle between the sexes seem to flare up when Lacan argues against his own structuralist attitude:[63] Considering the death of the father in Dora's second dream, Lacan observes a tendency in the hysteric structure that is disturbing to him – hysterics are inclined to change the roles in analysis. The hysteric (woman) instead of the (male) analyst tries to become the one who is supposed to know. One might argue that Lacan sticks to gender stereotypes of female patients and male analysts here. The hysteric makes the man believe that the woman has knowledge he does not have. According to Lacan, this goes hand in hand with a female death wish towards the man. In Dora's case, this facet is symbolized by the father's death in her dream.[64] What does a woman know? Lacan puts it like this: She knows what is necessary for a man's *jouissance* but does not realize this is a way of castrating him.

In the late 1960s, Lacan again points to the castrated father, now conceived of as the castrated master signifier, S1. The symbolic father reveals himself to be imaginary, whereas the father of Freud's former hysteric patients was idealized in his symbolic potency.[65] For Lacan, the father is now nothing but

---

[60] See J. Lacan, *Le Séminaire. Livre VIII (1960-1961). Le transfer*. Paris: Éditions du Seuil, 2001, p. 288ff.

[61] J. Lacan, *Le Séminaire. Livre XI (1964). Les quatres concepts de la psychanalyse*. Paris: Éditions du Seuil, p. 38.

[62] Bruno, *Le père et ses noms*, p. 142.

[63] Elements of a structure gain meaning only through their position and not through an essential attribute. To regard oneself as male or female in such a strict structuralist sense would only be a question of one's place in the signifying chain. See also G. Deleuze, *Woran erkennt man den Strukturalismus?* Berlin: Merve, 1992, p. 15.

[64] J. Lacan, *Le Séminaire. Livre XVI (1968-1969). D'un Autre à l'autre*. Paris: Éditions du Seuil, p. 388.

[65] J. Lacan, *Le Séminaire. Livre XVII (1969-1970). L'envers de la psychanalyse*. Paris: Éditions du Seuil, 1991, p. 108.

a structural operator (S1) who passes on the castration by which he, too, has been afflicted.⁶⁶ There are consequences for Lacan's view on Dora: To him, she is mainly interested not in the jewelry but in the box of her first dream, which hints at the fact that she knows how to enjoy.⁶⁷ She is keen to get the knowledge as a means of *jouissance* to serve the master's truth.⁶⁸ In the empty box at the apartment in her second dream, Dora finds a book containing the knowledge she is after: the truth about the sex.⁶⁹ Contrary to his former opinion, Lacan now doubts that the Oedipus complex is a useful tool for understanding the situation.⁷⁰

Lacan's handling of the signification of Dora's father during his teaching years reflects his changing ways of describing the functions associated with a father. There are some surprising facts in his reading of Dora's case; for instance, he does not point directly to a phallic connotation of Dora's early memory of sucking her thumb, and he ascribes a psychotic state to Dora when she is confronted with the collapse of her stabilizing phantasies. Lacan conceptualizes the father as a form of protection. In his interpretation of Dora's psychotic state, Lacan, unlike Freud, accentuates a protective function of the Name-of-the-Father against the mother's grasping desire.

In the 1960s, Lacan's theoretical frame of reference moves from a (phallus-oriented) theory of desire to a theory of *jouissance*. This shift, which is not limited to his reasoning about the father, goes in parallel with another transformation of his approach: The father as such becomes less important from the early 1960s, as Lacan ceases to believe in the figure of the father as a stable anchor of symbolic order.⁷¹ In both the desire-oriented and the *jouissance*-oriented theory, the paternal functions in reality, in phantasy and in transference are broken down into separate aspects: Real, imaginary and symbolic fathers have to be distinguished; other elements, like the Name-of-the-Father, the metaphor of the father, the big Other, O, the object, little o, and the signifier S1, have to be taken into consideration, too. As abstract forms they represent special features which might, but need not, interfere with the father's function.

---

⁶⁶ P. Verhaeghe, 'Enjoyment and Impossibility: Lacan's Revision of the Oedipus Complex', in: *sic 6. Jacques Lacan and the Other Side of Psychoanalysis. Reflections on Seminar XVII*. Durham, London: Duke University Press, 2006, p. 43.
⁶⁷ Lacan, *L'envers de la psychanalyse*, p. 109.
⁶⁸ Ibid., p. 110.
⁶⁹ Ibid., p. 111.
⁷⁰ Ibid., p. 113.
⁷¹ See also J.-A. Miller, 'The Other without the Other', see http://www.lacan.com/actuality/jacques-alain-miller-the-other-without-other/ (accessed on 30-6-2017).

In Lacan's work, the issue of the signification of Dora's father is closely interwoven with questions of her position as a woman with a lesbian desire. Unlike Freud in the clinical treatment, Lacan reading Freud's text realizes Dora's gender-related question. The role he ascribes to the father in his first references to Dora's case resembles the one Freud describes in the Oedipus complex.[72] The concept of the phallus as a signifier functioning beyond concrete fathers and the later idea of a woman's knowledge of *jouissance* are very useful elements to describe in detail Dora's search for her gender role[73] – only their connection with the father tends to fade. The model of the Oedipus complex finally fails to explain the details of Dora's gender choice. This is why one could say that her search points to an area beyond the father.

IV

In the beginning, Freud's and Lacan's approaches are comparable in that both see Dora's relationship with her father within an Oedipal frame, but overall there are more differences than similarities, with Lacan finally leaving the Oedipal frame. Freud had to cast off Philipp Bauer's influence, a problem Lacan of course never had. Lacan looked at the text only and tried to find the place the father occupied in Dora to explain her symptoms and her sexual orientation. Freud on the other hand was not prepared to first and foremost explore the issue of Dora's gender.

At least two aspects highlight the difference between Freud's and Lacan's approaches. The first aspect concerns the social function of the father. Freud and his hysteric patients lived in a time when the father figure had already started to lose its self-evident importance in the family. But in Dora's case, Freud thought she had only started the treatment due to her father's influence, and he was oblivious to the fact that the father might be part of the problem. In contrast, Lacan in an early text reacted to the social fact of paternal decline and pointed to diminished forms of the paternal *imago*.[74] Taking into account

---

[72] One can distinguish three versions of the Oedipus complex in Lacan's early approach: a classic version where the idealization of the father allows the child to leave the close attachment to the mother, a second version in which the decline of the paternal imago corresponds with a compensatory strong attachment to the mother and a third version with a humiliated figure of the father. See also, M. Zafiropoulos, *Du père mort au déclin du père de famille. Où va la psychanalyse?* Paris: Presses Universitaires de France, 2014, p. 66.

[73] On some problems with Lacan's concept of feminity (i.e. his idea of Medea being the true woman), see ibid., p. 139ff.

[74] J. Lacan, 'Les complexes familiaux dans la formation de l'individu. Essai d'analyse d'une fonction en psychologie (1938)', in: *Autres Écrits*. Paris: Le Seuil, 2001, p. 56. The *imago* of the father stands for imaginary effects the figure of the father has in social as well as individual contexts.

the moral and physical weakness of Dora's father, Philipp Bauer is a perfect example of the decline of the paternal figure in the patriarchal family.[75] Freud remains sympathetic or at least neutral towards his patient's father, whereas Lacan clearly marks his moral weakness in his first references to the case. As the later-born and *après coup*, Lacan can take into account different aspects of the father's role over the following years. He soon changes his nostalgic view of the father's vanishing *imago* in the family and develops structuralist tools to describe changing social realities,[76] in this case the reduced social impact of paternal authority.

The second aspect concerns gender roles that have undergone far-reaching transformations over the past century. Freud's inability to sufficiently consider Dora's lesbian desire has to be understood in the context of the fact that women's liberation and the increasing social acceptance of homosexual relationships are cultural achievements of the 20th century in some western countries. Lacan's psychoanalytic quasi-mathematical formalizations, on the other hand, allow describing changing gender structures. Over the past decades, LGBTIQ groups have raised the profile of their cause, and one might wonder whether Dora today would find herself advocating for the inclusion of all genders and accuse Mr K., Freud or her father of glossing over the domestic violence she experienced. Today, the discussion of reports of sexual assault mainly focuses on facts in reality.[77] On the other hand, though, one has to admit that Freud, unlike his contemporaries, was already tackling the difficult question of daughters reporting their fathers, other close relatives or friends for having molested, seduced or sexually abused them when they were younger. And it was Freud's way of dealing with the signification of Dora's father that opened up a way of actually taking into account a broad variety of different unconscious aspects that shape the experiences of daughters and fathers up to this day.

---

[75] P. Verhaeghe, *Says Who? The struggle for authority in a market-based society*. London: Scribe Publications, 2017.
[76] Zafiropoulos points to the fact that Lacan abandoned the theory of the decline of the father's *imago* when he turned away from the sociologist Émile Durkheim under the influence of Claude Levi-Strauss. Zafiropoulos, *Du père mort*, p. 89.
[77] As an example, see H. Dressing et al., 'Sexual abuse of minors within the Catholic Church and other institutions', in *Neuropsychiatrie* 17 (2017/2), pp. 45-55.

From Dora to Conchita:
Recent Views on Gender and Sexuality
in Psychoanalysis

Ilka Quindeau

Why Dora? Freud's famous Dora case study, 'Fragment of an Analysis of a Case of Hysteria',[1] has attracted more comment than almost any of his other case studies. Freud made no attempt to paper over the cracks in it, and instead left inconsistencies and unanswered questions to speak for themselves.[2] His account of psychological vagaries is so graphic, and his deployment of theoretical approaches is so precise, that decades later it is still eminently rewarding to return to this material in order to compare contrast it with new views on the subject. Since it was published in 1905, countless articles, collections, and monographs have appeared in response to the Dora case, notably by American and French psychoanalysts. The Dora case has been discussed from every conceivable perspective, by advocates of intersubjective, relational, or Lacanian psychoanalysis as well as from the perspective of treatment technique and trauma comprehension.[3]. Engaging with the unsettling aspects of the case and appreciating their implications is a constant challenge.[4] Hence my question: What exactly is it that still makes this case unsettling?

Dora's treatment lasted only three months, taking place in the fall of 1900, shortly after the original publication of *The Interpretation of Dreams* (1900).[5] The account of the case was originally planned as a continuation and extension of that work, the reason why two of Dora's dreams take center stage. Today, however, the critical reception accorded to the Dora case focuses less on Freud's interpretation of her dreams than on the underlying theory of femininity to which the failure of his treatment is frequently ascribed. Gender and sexuality are still central identity markers in a largely heteronormative society that demands clear-cut gendered distinctions. In psychoanalysis, these two issues – gender identity and sexual identity – are connected, rather amalgamated, within the

---
[1] S. Freud, 'A Fragment of an Analysis of a Case of Hysteria' (1905 [1901]), *SE* 7, pp. 3-122.
[2] See, P. Mahony, 'Freud's Unadorned and Unadorable: A Case History terminable and Interminable', in: *Psychoanalytic Inquiry* 25 (2005), pp. 27-44.
[3] See, S.S. Lewine, 'Prologue', in: *Psychoanalytic Inquiry* 25 (2005), pp. 1-4, etc.
[4] See, V. King, 'Faszination und Anstößigkeit: Der "Fall Dora" im Entstehungs- und Veränderungsprozeß der Psychoanalyse', in: *Psyche* 60 (2006), pp. 978-1004.
[5] S. Freud, *The Interpretation of Dreams* (1900), *SE* 4-5.

Oedipal conflict. The Oedipal conflict inscribes societal structure principles such as gender dichotomy into the psychic structure of the individual, while genital primacy – the definition of polymorphous sexuality as "fore-pleasure" and its subordination to the dominance of the genital – cements the principle of heteronormativity.

My thesis is that the failure of Dora's treatment has to do with Freud's heteronormative approach. Dora resisted this approach by discontinuing the analysis, which was tantamount to a refusal to accommodate herself to Freud's theory of femininity. In doing so, she was also challenging heteronormativity as a societal imperative. To set this out in more detail, I intend to situate the case history in the context of the early development of psychoanalysis at the crucial point where Freud famously changed his theoretical tack and relinquished his seduction theory to make way for the formulation of the Oedipal conflict. This was equivalent to replacing the primacy of the Other with the primacy of the subject.

From seduction theory to Oedipus conflict

"I no longer believe in *my neurotica*".[6] This much-quoted sentence that Freud wrote to his friend Wilhem Fliess in September 1897 marks a central turning point in the history of psychoanalysis: the so-called 'abandonment' of seduction or trauma theory. Rarely in the academic historiography of psychoanalysis has there been such an overwhelming degree of unanimity as there is about Freud's relinquishment of his seduction theory. It is regarded by analysts of all persuasions and theoretical convictions as the decisive breakthrough in the evolution of psychoanalysis as a theory in its own right.

What does this theory say? Unlike the medical theories prevalent at the time, Freud did not trace hysteria back to 'degenerative' factors of a hereditary and/or somatic nature. Instead, he proposed a trauma model in which retrospective psychic engagement with an event – and not the event itself – plays the decisive etiological role. This insight is expressed pointedly in the famous dictum: "*Hysterics suffer mainly from reminiscences.*"[7] Here Freud turns his back on the traditional medical concept of trauma with its distinction between (objective) event and (subjective) experience, replacing it with an intricately interwoven dialectical relationship between 'inside' and 'outside,' 'subject' and 'object'.

---

[6] *The Complete Letters of Sigmund Freud to Wilhelm Fliess 1887–1904*, J.M. Masson (Ed.). Cambridge, MA: The Belknap Press of Harvard University Press, 1985, p. 264.
[7] J. Breuer & S. Freud, *Studies on Hysteria* (1895), SE 2, p. 7.

He sees neurotic symptoms as originating in the attempt to ward off insupportable, intensely embarrassing thoughts or feelings. These he traces back to sexual experiences in early childhood, i.e. prior to pubescence, of the kind reported by his hysterical female patients in therapy. These were accounts of sexual or erotic relations, from seductions all the way up to violent sexual interference inflicted on them by adult caregivers, relatives, teachers of both sexes, and older children. Freud saw these experiences as an essential factor in the onset of neurosis, marveling however at the frequency of these events (surely there could hardly have been so many perverted adults around) and the regularity with which they figured in the life histories of his hysterical female patients.

Assailed by doubts about this regularity, Freud made an important decision. He freed himself of the "overestimation of reality and the underestimation of fantasy"[8] and began interpreting the accounts of his female patients not so much as descriptions of real sexual experiences but as manifestations of unconscious fantasies.

Today we may be inclined to ask whether by revoking his seduction theory so unequivocally and positing such a sharp distinction between fantasy and reality Freud was not in fact throwing out the baby with the bath water. This theoretical volte-face not only has repercussions on Freud's theory of femininity, it in fact represents a paradigm shift of the kind defined by Thomas Kuhn, a revision of views involving far-reaching modifications to the theoretical and methodological persuasions he had formerly espoused.

Freud formulated his concept of the Oedipus complex more or less at the same time as he jettisoned his seduction theory in the context of his own self-analysis:[9]

> "A single idea of genuine value dawned on me. I have found, in my own case too, [the phenomenon of] being in love with my mother and jealous of my father, and I now consider it a universal event in early childhood (…). If this is so, we can understand the gripping power of *Oedipus Rex*, in spite of all the objections that reason raises against the presupposition of fate (…). Everyone in the audience was once a budding Oedipus in fantasy and each recoils in horror from the dream fulfillment here transplanted into reality, with the full quantity of repression which separates his infantile state from his present one."[10]

---

[8] S. Freud, 'The Aetiology of Hysteria' (1896), *SE* 3, pp. 187-221, p. 204.
[9] See, letters No. 139, 141, 142 to Wilhelm Fliess, September and October 1897, *The Complete Letters*, pp. 264-273.
[10] Ibid., p. 272.

Jean Laplanche gave in 1987 a detailed critical account of the theory – historical connection between the abandonment of seduction theory and the formulation of the Oedipal conflict.[11] The withdrawal of seduction theory relegates the external traumatization of the subject to the background. In its place we have the significance of psychic reality and fantasy. The problem is the substitution of reality by fantasy. Put succinctly, we can describe this as a de-historicization and a mythologization of psychoanalytic theory. From now on, Freud regards the universality of Oedipal fantasies as a phylogenetic legacy. In Freud's theoretical development, the demise of seduction theory turns fantasy and reality into opposing forces. This tendency is doubly true of Freud's successors. By understanding them as an archaic legacy, Freud lifts the primal structure-forming fantasies – on the primal scene, castration, or seduction – out of the concrete life history of the individual and establishes them in the realm of mythology. Thus a constitutive concept (unconscious fantasy) is severed from its biographical roots. It fails to acquire a genuinely psychoanalytic foundation that connects reality with fantasy and conceives of fantasy as an engagement with biographical experiences, a process structured by existing societal schemas: primal scene, castration, Oedipus.

The low valuation of reality and overvaluation of universal fantasies

In his treatment of Dora, as set down in the case history, we can identify the theoretical and practical consequences of Freud's new withdrawal from the primacy of the Other. I take the evidence for this contention *pars pro toto* from the following aspects of the case: the status accorded to the actual instance of sexual interference by Herr K.; Freud's insistence on theoretical concepts rather than a joint-search for subjective significance; and Freud's acting-out in transference.

In his revocation of seduction theory, Freud was proud of having liberated himself from the "*overvaluation* of reality" and his "*low valuation* of phantasy".[12] But the case history points out the problems that this involves, attesting to the overestimation of the concept of universal Oedipal conflict in its heteronormative version. Freud appears to take Dora's actual experiences (sexual interference by Herr K.) less seriously. Against the backdrop of imputed Oedipal desires, he interprets her revulsion as a defense. Freud's response to the sexual incident is to pathologize Dora's reaction rather than acknowledge the physical violence involved. Dora's revulsion at the kiss Herr K. forces on her is interpreted as

---

[11] J. Laplanche, *New Foundations for Psychoanalysis*. Oxford: Basil Blackwell, 1989, pp. 207ff.
[12] Freud, 'The Aetiology of Hysteria', p. 204 (footnote added 1924).

hysterical: "Without hesitation, indeed without exception, I would consider any person who largely or exclusively experiences feelings of disgust when an occasion for sexual excitement presents itself to be hysterical."[13] Seduction theory had set out in plain terms the fact that actual sexual assault can result in trauma or be processed as a trauma. But this insight disappears entirely from Dora's case history. Fantasy and the engagement with fantasy turn pathogenic, appearing more or less divorced from factual reality. Whereas the earlier trauma concept focused essentially on the joint effect of factual and psychic reality, event and fantasy, Dora's case history shows us Freud turning away from this notion.

What we have instead is the 'traditional' imbalance of power between doctor and patient: the power of scientific definition and of hermeneutic interpretation replaces the primacy of the Other. Freud constantly insinuates that Dora is in love with Herr K., seeing this as the expression of an Oedipal conflict that she has failed to come to terms with. He interprets her conscious 'no' as an unconscious 'yes':

> "The 'no' one hears from the patient after one has presented his conscious perception with a repressed thought for the first time only registers the repression and its decisive character only means, as it were, its strength. If one takes this 'no' not as the expression of an impartial judgement, of which the patient is not in fact capable, disregards it, and continues the work, proofs will soon appear that 'no' in such a case signifies the desired 'yes'."[14]

Naturally, one can only concur with Freud's insight that repressed, forbidden wishes will indeed appear alien to the analysand, which means that initially he/she will be inclined to deny them. But this cannot be a justification for continuing to impute such desires without even considering the eventuality that one's own hypothesis might be at fault. True, Freud registers Dora's admiration and affection for Frau K., reporting Dora's praise for the "adorable white body in accents more appropriate to a lover than to a defeated rival".[15] From the perspective of his heteronormative assumptions, Freud interprets this merely as an indication of Ida's 'latent homosexuality' and attaches no further significance to it, thus enabling him to adhere to his hypothesis of Dora being in love with Herr K. An even clearer revelation of this heteronormativity is to be found in

---

[13] Freud, 'Fragment', p. 29.
[14] Ibid., p. 59.
[15] Ibid., p. 62.

Freud's assessment that she could have regained her health via "marriage and normal sexual intercourse".[16]

Dora's case history was the first to bring home to Freud the significance of transference and countertransference, in which he himself identified as one of the causes for the failure of his treatment. An initial reinterpretation in this direction came from Lacan in 1951,[17] from whom Freud's unconscious identification with Mr K. prompted the far-reaching insight that countertransference precedes transference, thus emphasizing the primacy of the Other. Without due attentiveness to the dynamics of transference and countertransference, Freud was unable to recognize the central role Dora accorded to him in her first dream and equally unable to hear, as King puts it, the "relational messages"[18] contained in that same dream. He was just as impervious to his negative countertransference, which manifested itself in massive disparagements and the assessment of Dora's desperate thoughts of suicide as a "Selbstmordkomödie" ('suicide comedy').[19] In this case study, Steven Marcus sees Freud as a kind of (Ibsenian) truth fanatic, acting more like a scientist than a therapist towards a patient caught up in some Victorian family drama. Thus Dora had no chance of figuring as the author in Freud's version of her life history. Instead of allowing Dora to appropriate her own story, Freud took possession of it himself and left her dispossessed.[20]

The significance and function that Freud ascribed to Dora's symptoms determined the technique he used. Herr K.'s assault repeated itself symbolically in the analytic situation: Freud 'penetrated' Dora with his interpretations. Emily Kuriloff refers to this as transferential/countertransferential 'body talk'.[21] Dora speaks through her body because she cannot obtain a response in any other way. But Freud reduces Dora's body language to accord with his theories and normative presuppositions and fails to explore the different levels of significance operative therein. Thus in practical fact he remained bogged down in the body-soul dualism that in his theories he had long since overcome.

---

[16] Ibid., p. 79.
[17] J. Lacan, 'Intervention sur le transfert' (1951), *Ecrits*. Paris: Seuil 1966, pp. 215-226.
[18] See, King, 'Faszination und Anstößigkeit'.
[19] In the *Standard Edition*, "Selbstmordkomödie" is translated with "pretence at suicide"; S. Freud, 'Fragment', p. 33.
[20] S. Marcus, 'Freud und Dora. Roman, Geschichte, Krankengeschichte', in: *Psyche* 28 (1974), pp. 32-79.
[21] E. Kuriloff, 'What's going on with Dora. An interpersonal perspective', in: *Psychoanalytic Inquiry* 25 (2005), pp. 71-83.

From Dora to Conchita: new challenges for psychoanalytic theory-formation

Over a hundred years later, in 2014, Conchita Wurst won the 59th Eurovision Song Contest with an overwhelming majority of votes. She was chosen by a jury and 120 million viewers from 26 countries. By choosing the pseudonym Conchita Wurst, the Austrian singer Thomas Neuwirth set out to show that gender is '*wurs(ch)t*' (colloquial German for 'irrelevant'). It is of no importance and has no role to play. The interesting thing about this winning act seems to me to be the fact that this is no ordinary drag queen. He does not simply use travesty to impersonate a woman, substituting femininity for masculinity. He lets both femininity and masculinity stand side-by-side. In his artificial persona he combines male and female, the most obvious instance being the full beard plus the female silhouette. This also extends to his pseudonym: *conchita* (little shell) is used colloquially in Spanish to refer to the female genitals, while *Wurst* (sausage) stands for the male phallus.

This enactment challenges our visual habits. We can see it as a critique of the heteronormativity still underlying psychoanalytic theory. The normative conceptions of identity encountered in psychoanalysis have a long history and astonishingly have rarely been a subject for reflection, which is odd, to say the least, in a profession that has dedicated itself to self-reflection. The question that poses itself here is whether this normativity is unavoidably inscribed into the theories or whether other, non-normative readings are possible. With regard to the formative principles behind sexuality and gender, the concept of Oedipal conflict is of crucial significance in psychoanalytic theory-formation. In its powerfully influential variant, the Oedipus complex, Freud binds up the development of sexual orientation with the acquisition of gender identity, a conception that has lost none of its impact in mainstream psychoanalysis to this day. In fact, however, this amalgamation between sexual orientation and gender is neither inescapable nor particularly plausible. It is a product of heteronormativity. In this vein, Judith Butler criticizes the insistence on the development of binary gender identity as a melancholic process that requires the aberrant love of the same-sex parent in order to identify with him/her.[22] Before that, O'Connor and Ryan had problematized the substitution relation between identification and desire in the traditional Oedipal conflict.[23] This conflict, they insist, is based on the hardly very compelling assumption of heterosexual complementarity as

---

[22] J. Butler, 'Melancholy Gender/Refused Identification', in: *The Psychic Life of Power: Theories in Subjection*. Stanford, CA: Stanford University Press, 1997, pp. 132-150.
[23] N. O'Connor & J. Ryan, *Wild Desires and Mistaken Identities: Lesbianism and Psychoanalysis*. London: Virago, 1993.

a necessary principle in the structuring of desire. Jessica Benjamin reformulates this relation by conceiving of identification as the precondition for desire.[24] She thus indicates a way of conceptualizing homosexual desire as non-pathological. The price for this is that desire no longer has the central, primary status accorded to it in Freudian psychoanalysis. Eva Poluda-Korte, another author writing in German, discusses the determination of the relation between identification and object-love, conceptualizing a 'lesbian complex' traditionally referred to as a negative Oedipus complex, the working-through of which can lead either to a homo- or to a heterosexual orientation.[25]

In recent years, published accounts of analytic treatment have increasingly been penned by authors who do not share these normative notions of identity.[26] Nevertheless, the underlying heteronormative theory is still very much with us, and there has been little in the way of explicit, systematic revision.[27] Against this background, I should like to reformulate the traditional concept of Oedipal conflict in an attempt to release it from heteronormative constrictions and rigid conceptualization.

Why do I adhere to the concept of the Oedipal conflict instead of relinquishing it together with all the problematic versions of it that have come down to us? Though, Oedipal conflict no longer plays such a central role in present-day psychoanalysis as it did in Freud's day, it is still crucially significant in the structuring of sexual complexion and personality. At the termination of the Oedipal conflict stands the recognition of otherness and difference, which in mainstream psychoanalysis is equated with the acknowledgement of bisexuality and heterosexuality, although as I have been trying to show, this is anything but a compelling conclusion. The aim of the termination is not to acquire an unambiguous identity clearly set off from the Other. In a more extended sense one might rather describe the aim as the development of tolerance for ambiguity, meaning the capacity to let differences and uncertainties stand side-by-side. Identity formations are not necessarily binary and heteronormative, they can be open and fluid enough to encompass the non-identical and let both male and female, homo- and heterosexuality, exist side by side. Though Freud restricted

---

[24] J. Benjamin, 'Sameness and Difference: Toward an "Overinclusive" Model of Gender Development', in: *Psychoanalytic Inquiry* 15 (1995), pp. 125-142.

[25] E. Poluda-Korte, 'Der "lesbische Komplex". Das homosexuelle Tabu und die Weiblichkeit', in: E.-M. Alves (Ed.), *Stumme Liebe. Der "lesbische Komplex" in der Psychoanalyse*. Freiburg: Kore 1993, pp. 73-32.

[26] Cf. the highly instructive volume by A. Lemma & P. Lynch, *Sexualities. Contemporary psychoanalytical perspectives*. London: Routledge, 2015.

[27] N. Barden, 'Disrupting Oedipus: the legacy of the Sphinx', A. Lemma & P. Lynch (Eds.), *Sexualities*, pp. xxx-xxxx; B. Möller & G. Romer, 'Geschlechtsdysphorie', in: *Praxis der Kinderpsychologie und Kinderpsychiatrie* 63 (2014), pp. 431-436.

his statement to the female case, what he said about the Oedipal conflict – i.e., that it could never be completely overcome – is of course true of all individuals. Oedipal conflict does not produce static, unchangeable solutions but is worked through time and again in the course of a life. This process can thus culminate indifferent gender identities or sexual orientations. This lifelong dynamism and mutability of the unconscious psychic conflict seems to me a very good reason to uphold the concept of Oedipal conflict while modifying it in such a way as to avoid heteronormativity.

My reformulation of Oedipal conflict takes its bearings from Jean Laplanche's general seduction theory,[28] a milestone in the recent history of psychoanalysis. He locates the origins of the unconscious and the sexual in a social situation, the relationship between child and adult. The child responds to the 'enigmatic messages' of the adult with the development of its unconscious, its sexuality, and its gender. This process culminates in the Oedipal conflict, in which the child psychically appropriates its desires and its gender.

First, however, I shall discuss the Freudian concept of 'constitutional bisexuality.' It provides interesting potential for an open, fluid, and biological (bodily) concept of gender. I find this last point particularly important because open concepts are frequently criticized for being located on the social or psychic plane without any physical foundation. I indicate why (biological) sex is also a construct, i.e. composed of various individual factors. Instead of the word 'core' I believe the metaphorical terms 'envelope' or 'container' to be more apposite in discussing gender identity.

Physical bisexuality provides the potential for multiple gender identifications. This casts doubt on psychoanalytic theories of the development of gender identity that, while they proceed from early identifications with father *and* mother, still consider it unavoidable in terms of psychic health for these various identifications to be replaced by an unambiguous, single-sex identity.

'Constitutional bisexuality' and multiple gender identifications

Challenging gender dichotomy is not new in psychoanalysis. As early as his lecture on femininity Freud emphasizes: "When you meet a human being, the first distinction you make is 'male or female?' And you are accustomed to making that distinction with unhesitating certainty."[29] He goes on to say that anatomical science only shares this certainty up to a certain point, because male features

---

[28] Laplanche, *New Foundations for Psychoanalysis*.
[29] S. Freud, 'Lecture XXXIII. Femininity', *New Introductory Lectures on Psycho-Analysis* (1933), *SE* 22, p. 112-135, p. 113.

are discernible in women's bodies and vice versa, "as though an individual is not a man or a woman but always both, just so much more of the one than the other."[30] Though Freud's remarks on masculinity and femininity are among the most controversial passages in his entire oeuvre and phallic monism – the theory that possessing or not possessing a male sex organ is the key to psychosexual development – has rightly been rejected, his 'constitutional bisexuality' can only be regarded as a seminal concept in the history of psychoanalytic theory. Physical masculinity and femininity are located on a continuum rather than being sharply distinguished from one another. Crucially important to my mind is the fact that Freud directly anchors this bisexual predisposition on the physical plane.

A distinction needs to be made between this biological bisexuality and the psychic bisexuality deriving from the presence of male and female traits engendered by identification processes with mother and father. Although Freud remained convinced of the significance of bisexuality, he never systematized the concept, and many of his successors (male and female) disagreed with him on the point, replacing the notion with the idea of gender identity, usually conceptualized as innate. It is tempting to speculate whether this move toward disambiguation may be connected with the increasing significance of sex/gender as a structural category in modern societies.

In the course of gender deconstruction in the social sciences and particularly in gender studies, the concept of constitutional bisexuality can be drawn upon to overcome a dichotomous, binary concept of gender. At this point I should like to discuss the present mainstream psychoanalytic theory on the development of gender identity. It was proposed by the American analyst Robert Stoller in the 1960s. He worked extensively with transgender individuals and penned a number of important publications on so-called perversions.[31] His theory can best be illustrated with the following diagram:

---

[30] Ibid., p. 114.
[31] See, R. Stoller, *Sex and Gender. On the Development of Masculinity and Femininity*. Vol.1. New York: Science House, 1968; R. Stoller, *Perversion: The Erotic Form of Hatred*. New York: Pantheon, 1975; R. Stoller, Robert, *Sex and Gender. The Transsexual Experiment*. Vol. 2. New York: Aronson, 1976.

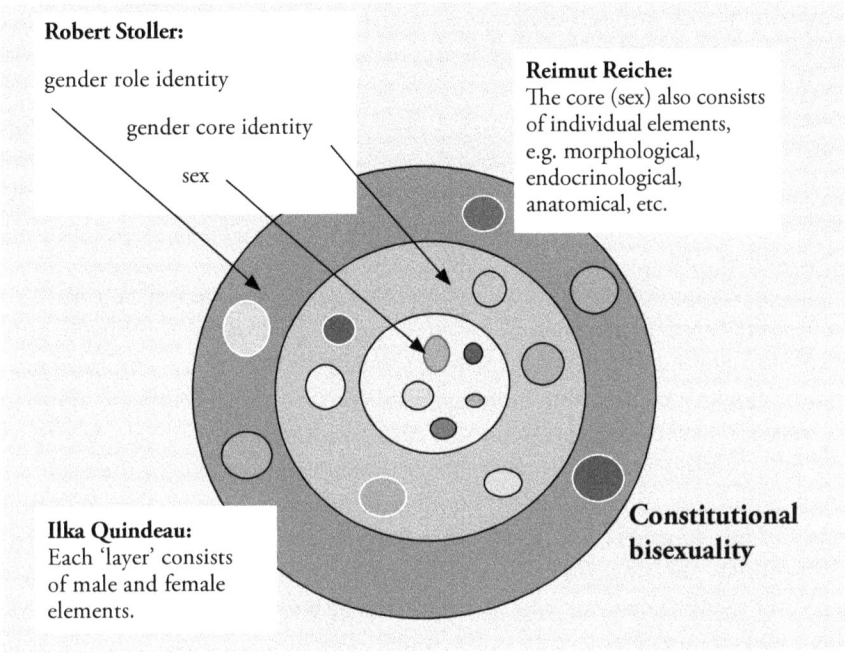

Constitutional bisexuality after Stoller, Reiche, and Quindeau

The concept of bisexuality is bound up with gender dichotomy, which is probably why it rarely figures in gender research. To sidestep this connection, it could be replaced by the notion of constitutional gender diversity. The epithet 'constitutional' is especially important here as it encompasses the somatic (sex) and not merely the psychic or psychosocial dimension (gender).

Diversity begins on the physical plane (sex). Biological sex itself is a composite and by no means only a 'core' of the kind referred to by Stoller in his concept of 'core gender identity.' Even today, however, the idea of core gender identity has remained a largely unchallenged standard concept. What does the concept imply?

Stoller posits a core, surrounded by two concentric circles or layers. The inner core is equivalent to biological sex. It is encircled by a layer that is either isomorphic or anisomorphic and itself forms another core: core gender identity. In its turn, this second core is encircled by gender role identity, which stands for the whole panoply of gender-related self/object representations, plus societal conventions and norms. Shortly after the publication of this model, Reimut Reiche deconstructed the core, revealing it as a composite and pointing out that with his use of the term 'core identity,' Stoller was not referring to empirical reality (though the term is frequently used to do precisely that) but to a scientific concept.[32] His main criticism was that Freud's bisexuality had been left out of account and that the development of this core was conceived of as being 'free of conflict.' From the perspective of general seduction theory and the many gender-related messages emanating both from a child's reference persons and various societal ascriptions, we can only agree. By contrast, the idea of isomorphic/anisomorphic identity formation appears both simplistic and reductionist.

Contrary to received opinion, biological sex is not a monolithic entity but a composite construct made up of various elements. Biological sex refers not only to the genitals but encompasses other factors as well: anatomical, chromosomal, morphological, endocrinological, etc. This 'constructedness' appears to me to be crucial. Societal consensus (in this case, scientific and medical consensus) dictates the dimensions that are to be regarded as constitutive for the sex of an individual. This consensus is by no means immutable across all periods and cultures but depends on such things as diagnostic and technological progress. Accordingly, referring to *Geschlecht* (sex and gender) as a construct relates not only to the psychological or social aspects but also to the biology of the matter. Eloquent examples of this are to be found, say, in intersexual individuals in whom phenomenological sex differs from their chromosomal complexion, a discrepancy revealed by the recent progress in genetic engineering.

Any attempt to elaborate a model for this will necessarily involve a thoroughgoing revision and extension of the metaphor of the three 'layers.' In Stoller's model, these layers foster the impression that the individual strata of biological, psychic, and social gender exist independently of one another. The model is largely resistant to the idea of interrelations between the different planes. There is no way of identifying how gender-related relationship experiences are inscribed into the body or, vice versa, how physical sexual experiences affect experiences in relationships. To find an appropriate way of representing such interactional relations between the various levels, I propose taking Freud's concept of constitutional bisexuality as a starting point and positing various ratios of 'male' and 'female' elements as existing not only between the different layers but also within those three layers themselves. Biological sex, for example, is constituted by various anatomical, morphological or endocrinological features that are by no means unequivocally 'male' or 'female' but contain both male and female elements. This diversity is apparent in each human individual, not only at the level of co-existent 'male' and 'female' behaviors but also in such things

---

[32] R. Reiche, 'Gender ohne Sex. Geschichte, Funktion und Funktionswandel des Begriffs "Gender"', in: *Psyche* 51 (1997), pp. 926-957.

as specific hormone ratios or physical features attributed to one gender or the other in a reductionist way (i.e. high testosterone levels are 'male,' body curves are 'female.'). Accordingly, there seems to be little point in attempting to regard biological sex as something cut and dry. It would be more convincing to think of it in terms of different ratios operating at both one and the same level and also between those levels. This would give the concept of gender *diversity* greater definition, not only as an 'idealistic' category, which it is frequently thought to be, but also at a concrete, material level fully embracing the physical dimension.

For a psychoanalytic understanding of gender identity I believe that the three-layer model is inappropriate. It should be replaced by the metaphor of an envelope or container enclosing the various conscious and unconscious aspects of masculinity and femininity which in different ratios in the various somatic, psychic, and social dimensions. Our culture encodes sex/gender in binary terms. Accordingly it has only two different envelopes or containers. But they can certainly contain identical, or at least similar, things. The envelope or container metaphor also points up the fact that gender identity is not something uniform or monolithic but is made up of various individual male and female aspects, some of them contradictory or even irreconcilable. With this metaphor – envelope or container – I propose a different view of gender identity from Robert Stoller's, whose concept of gender identity as a 'core' has underlain psychoanalytic discourse more or less explicitly over the last 40 years or so. My model is an inversion of Stoller's. Whereas Stoller proceeds from a core as an internal structure and focuses on the layers around this core, my perspective moves from a visible outward surface to the variegated aspects behind it. From a psychoanalytic perspective, container content and content diversity are much more interesting than the binary coding surface, which specifically serves a societal structure function. Proceeding from the distinction made by Freud, I should thus like to advocate that psychoanalytic thinking should move away from cultural dichotomy and embrace a diversification of the sexes.

Multiple gender identifications
The approximately 50 gender categories encountered on Facebook and in other social media suggest that gender identifications are arbitrary processes left to the discretion of individuals. From the viewpoint of the theory of general seduction, however, such self-constructions are hardly conceivable. Laplanche emphasized that children are not actively identified 'with' but 'by' adults on the basis of the ambient bisexually structured societies in place before the individual subject arrives on the scene. The passive form, i.e. ascription, is

crucial in Laplanche's thinking. It turns gender (like desire) into something that individuals do not have at their disposal as autonomous beings. It is however not entirely structured from the outside via ascription, it originates in the complex interplay between the ego and the Other as the result of psychic engagement with ascription in all its variety. Like all psychic work, this process takes place unconsciously and of course cannot be intentionally influenced. In addition, the ascriptions with regard to gender identity cannot all be expected to point in the same direction. First, there are always a number of people identifying the child as male or female. Secondly, these ascriptions take place both consciously and unconsciously. Thus in each person there is a whole bundle of ascriptions encompassing both male and female features.

Reimut Reiche refers to these gender ascriptions as 'enigmatic messages'.[33] This again is a concept coined by Laplanche. The unconscious messages emanate from the adult and are directed at the child, who must decipher, translate, and come to terms with them psychically. This, I feel, is a very accurate description of this complex, multi-faceted process. The child is not entirely passive in its exposure to the ascriptions, but rather must deal with them. And this process is not restricted to early childhood but continues, in principle, throughout a person's life.

A brief example may help to elucidate the point. When a mother says to her child: "You are Peter, a boy," the statement contains any number of gender-related ideas and expectations. One of them is whatever is understood to be a boy at a given time in a given society or culture. This is joined by all the mother's personal, subjective notions and experiences with men or masculinity in the course of her life, i.e. all her experiences with her father and brothers, plus the boys and men in the various stages of her life, all the way up to the father of her child. These experiences, whether largely positive or more negative and conflictual, will have an influence on the maleness of the son. This is true not only of the mother but also of the father and other important reference persons. All of them have been through different experiences with boys and men/masculinity and transpose those experiences – in the form of 'enigmatic messages' – into their interactions with the child. Laplanche calls this process 'intromission', a term designed to emphasize its urgent, inevitable character. Something is 'transmitted' to the child that it has to decipher and translate. In the course of this psychic process, the child's gender assignment takes shape in tune with society's pre-existent binary coding mechanism. Institutions like kindergarten and school play a crucial role, structuring and regulating the

---

[33] Ibid.

processes that constitute identity.[34] Intromissions and the psychic engagement with them influence the formation of the child's gendered body. Accordingly, biological sex does not exist independently of these inscriptions, nor is it prior to them.

A new-fledged father has come to my practice for counsel. He already has three sons and was very much hoping for a daughter, but the fourth child also turned out to be a son. At a conscious level, the baby has of course been brought up as a boy, but unconsciously the wishes bound up with a girl have been communicated to him subliminally. None of this need necessarily lead to psychic conflicts, let alone manifest disorders. These complex gender ascriptions are present in every person.

The majority of recent psychological theories assume that it is indispensable to develop an unambiguous, single-sex identity if our mental health is not to suffer. In 1984, Irene Fast proposed a theory of gender that is still widely espoused in mainstream psychoanalysis. The paradigm underlying her approach is differentiation. She contends that initially individuals are undifferentiated with respect to gender, so children's earliest experiences do not differ in a gender-specific way. In this early period, children experience themselves as 'over-inclusive'. Only at the age of about two years do children become aware of a gender difference. As a result, their experiences are then 're-gendered'. Notions of masculinity and femininity take shape, formulated and developed initially with reference to father and mother. Finally, a clearly demarcated, complexly structured feeling of self materializes. Taking a girl as an example, Fast describes this development as the emergence of a well-defined feeling of herself as a specifically female being, identifying with other women, experiencing herself in the relationship to them as specifically female, and developing a productive relationship to men, perceiving them in their maleness as independent of herself.[35] To acquire this well-defined dichotomous gender identity, children achieving an awareness of gender difference will deny their earlier over-inclusive representations and identifications as no longer compatible with their own gender. Donna Bassin criticizes the way Fast substitutes simple acceptance of reality for the rich, over-inclusive representations entertained previously.[36] She goes on to assert that Fast's epigenetic (and Piagetian) model of development ignores the fact that denied, rejected representations may retain their impact in

---

[34] See, M. Jäckle, S. Eck, M. Schnell & K. Schneider, *Doing Gender Discourse: Subjektivation von Mädchen und Jungen in der Schule*. Wiesbaden: Springer, 2016.
[35] I. Fast, *Gender Identity: A differentiation model*. Hillside NJ: Analytic Press, 1984, p. 25.
[36] D. Bassin, 'Beyond the He and She: Toward the reconciliation of masculinity and femininity in the post-oedipal female mind', *Journal of the American Psychoanalytical Association* 44 (1996), pp. 157-190.

the unconscious. She also takes issue with Fast's conceptualization of 'gender-inappropriate' attitudes that should be jettisoned in favor of a gender identity that squares with reality.[37] Fast's discussion conveys the impression that deciding on what is gender-appropriate or otherwise is invariably an unambiguous matter. Cultural change is completely left out of account. In every subjective account of development, conflict is invariably bound up, both culturally and individually, with these attempts at self-definition, and it recurs perennially in psychoanalysis. But here it is rigorously ignored. Ultimately, therefore, and in spite of her protestations to the contrary, Fast's approach is in fact indicative of a biological or essentialist understanding of gender.

The important thing to stress here is that the significance of gender identity is a cultural postulation, not an anthropological constant. Nor is dichotomous exclusiveness an imperative for development; we could equally well conceive of a species of gender assignment that permits male and female aspects to stand side-by-side.

Judith Butler describes the development of gender identity as a melancholy process.[38] Under the conditions dictated by binary coding, the diversity of gender identifications must yield to monosexual identity. In contrast to grief, melancholia has no awareness of loss. The losses of melancholia are unconscious. Precisely the same thing happens to gender identity in our culture. There is no mourning for the loss of a child's variegated gender identifications. On the contrary, acquisition of an unambiguous gender identity is celebrated as a step in the right developmental direction. At this point, I think it would be interesting to reflect on how one might accompany children in this development process without relegating loss to the unconscious. Perhaps mourning rituals might be beneficial.

From normative notions of identity to tolerance for ambiguity

My concept of 'tolerance for ambiguity' is designed to cast doubt on the normative line of development that leads to a total disambiguation of sex and sexuality, in other words to challenge its identitarian logic. Instead, I suggest understanding Oedipal conflict as a central locus for the psychic appropriation of difference and ambiguity.

Like Freud and Laplanche, I understand Oedipal conflict as a structural model. To my mind, the gender-specific manifestations proposed, say, by differential feminists, are problematic. By positing a specifically female Oedipus complex set off from the male variety they inevitably bolster the dominance of binary

---

[37] Ibid., p. 78ff.
[38] Butler, 'Melancholy Gender/Refused Identification'.

coding and hence of heteronormativity in our culture. If the Oedipal conflict is to remain significant in ongoing psychoanalytic theory formation, it can only do so in the form of a general structural model that leaves sufficient scope for both gender diversity and sexual diversity.

At this point, let me briefly recapitulate Freud's conceptualization of Oedipal conflict. Freud distinguished a 'positive' and a 'negative' form of the Oedipus complex that conjoin to constitute the fully-fledged complex.[39] The positive form adheres to the myth of Oedipus and links love of the other-sex parent with rivalry and death wishes vis-à-vis the same-sex parent. In its negative form we have love of the same-sex parent associated with rivalry vis-à-vis the other sex. The simultaneity of a homo- and heterosexual object choice – love for both the father and the mother – in the context of Oedipal conflict is possible because of the 'constitutional bisexuality' of the individual. Bisexuality refers not only to object choice but also to *gender*.

What we have here is a heteronormative model based on a dichotomous view of the sexes and on male-female parent couples. We need only recall the widespread phenomenon of single mothers/fathers or same-sex parents to realize that this does not adequately represent the reality of present-day family structures. The important thing about the model, however, is its triadic nature. Laplanche describes the Oedipal conflict as the Copernican revolution in a child's development.[40] Up to that point, the relational structure is dyadic. The pre-Oedipal child has dyadic relations to individual persons. It experiences itself as the hub of the world, similar in this to the Ptolemaic view of the universe. In the course of the Oedipal conflict, the child's relations gravitate from the dyad to the triad. The relations of the parents to one another and to siblings, friends, relatives, etc. take on psychic relevance for the child. This is a quantum leap in human development, though in some cases it never actually happens: there are adults who still consider themselves to be the hub of the universe.

The triadic relation structure can now be filled with other persons outside the customary nuclear family. All that is needed for the formation of psychic structure is a third person, regardless of gender or the degree of kinship.

Freud sees the upshot of the Oedipus complex in the establishment of sexual orientation and gender identity. Clinical experience and sexological research indicate, however, that it is by no means rare for changes in object choice to take place in the course of a lifetime. Instead of interpreting this as an indication

---

[39] S. Freud, 'The Dissolution of the Oedipus Complex' (1924), *SE* 19, pp. 171-179.
[40] Laplanche, *New Foundations for Psychoanalysis*; J. Laplanche, *Freud and the Sexual*. New York: International Psychoanalytic Books, 2011.

that the persons in question have been suppressing their 'authentic' proclivities, it is surely much more meaningful to assume that sexual orientation is not established once and for all in the framework of the Oedipus complex in early childhood or adolescence but rather that, like any other desire, its structure is the result of ongoing re-inscriptions. The Oedipal conflict can recur at various junctures in a person's life and find resolution in a variety of ways. With regard to gender identification and sexual orientation, these Oedipal resolutions are distinguished by their lifelong dynamics and their intrinsic mutability. The fluid, dynamic identities materializing in this way are not based on sharp delimitation from others but leave ample scope for the non-identical and the non-binary.

Conclusion

Perhaps the fascination of Dora's case has to do with the way it invites us to switch back and forth with our identifications. At times we adopt the analysand's position, at other times the analyst's. We feel an urge to grapple with Freud. In response to his account, we find ourselves saying, as in most case discussions: "I'd have done that quite differently." At all events, the Dora case confirms Freud's seminal status in psychoanalytic discourse, a figure we have no choice but to engage with. Engagement with this case history also opens our eyes to the normativity of the concepts and preliminary assumptions operative in Freud's approach. This heteronormativity is particularly striking in connection with his assumptions on femininity and sexual orientation. By no means rarely, his position on these identity issues is at odds with his theoretical views. Hardly any other sector of human behavior and experience is so susceptible to historical and cultural change. Taking the positive variant of Oedipal conflict as the key to the understanding of an analysand is an approach that is by no means restricted to Freud. Even today, this constellation is quite simply presumed to exist in the analysand, frequently without our even being aware of the fact. And yet it is crucial to inquire whether heterosexual love for the father is desire or defense, for, as the case of Dora indicates, it is often only too easy to classify something as pathological although this is not the case. For example, the assumption of the existence of Oedipal desires prompted Freud to interpret Dora's rejection of Herr K. as a defense and accordingly to declare it pathological, instead of understanding it as her response to sexual interference on K.'s part.

The problem with heteronormative assumptions is that they are so deeply ingrained in our culture and thus so apparently self-evident that they are very often no longer perceived to be hypotheses that may or may not be correct. Analysands like Dora and performers like Conchita Wurst draw our attention to the erroneous and problematic axiomaticity of heteronormative assumptions in psychoanalysis and therapy and indicate how inaccurate the binary coding of gender and sexuality can be.

The Case of Dora –
A Queer Perspective on Hysteria and Perversion

Esther Hutfless

Many feminists have regarded Dora – together with Anna O. and the young women from Sigmund Freud's study 'Psychogenesis of a Case of Female Homosexuality' – as heroines "of feminist protest against a psychoanalysis which was doing no more than reconfirming the prevailing sexual norms".[1] The feminist appropriation of the Freudian case studies as narratives about women's resistance to patriarchy and heteronormativity is closely linked with interpreting neurotic symptoms or perversion as subversive strategies against the hegemonial symbolic order. In addition, hysteria and perversion are criticized as discursive strategies within power relations, which produce and control specific subjects. They be allies of patriarchal, medical and heteronormative discourses. Is Dora – or the homosexual young woman of the *Psychogenesis* – a victim or a heroin? Are hysteria or perversion subversive or suppressive? There is no simple and definite answer to these questions. Jacques Derrida introduced the term 'undecidability' for those phenomena that do not "conform to either polarity of a dichotomy".[2] And Michel Foucault stated in *History of Sexuality*: "Where there is power, there is resistance, and yet, or rather consequently, this resistance is never in a position of exteriority in relation to power".[3] Power and resistance are intrinsically interwoven. For Foucault this entanglement is also innate to psychoanalysis itself:

> "It is very well to look back from our vantage point and remark upon the normalizing impulse in Freud; one can go on to denounce the role played for many years by the psychoanalytic institution; but the fact remains that in the great family of technologies of sex, which goes so far back into the history of the Christian West, of all those institutions that set out in the nineteenth century to medicalize sex, it was the one

---

[1] R. Bowlby, 'Still crazy after all these years', *Between Feminism and Psychoanalysis*, T. Brennan (Ed.). New York: Routledge, 1989, p. 45.
[2] J. Reynolds, 'Decision', J. Reynolds & J. Roffe (Eds.), *Understanding Derrida*. New York: Continuum, 2004, p. 46. The undecidable in Derrida's work has much more implications. See, J. H. Miller, *For Derrida*. New York: Fordham University Press, 2009, p. 17ff.
[3] M. Foucault, *The History of Sexuality. Volume I: An Introduction*. New York: Pantheon Books, 1978, p. 95.

that, up to the decade of the forties, rigorously opposed the political and institutional effects of the perversion-heredity-degenerescence system."[4]

And last no least, when assessing the famous case study of Dora, one should remember Freud's own words after treating Dora for three months only: in his *Prefatory Remarks* he reminds us, that "[i]t is not fair to expect from a single case more than it can offer".[5]

Thus, instead of offering another interpretation or re-reading of Dora's case, in this essay, I rather would like to address general questions, such as: How to deal with concepts that have such a long history in support of oppression? What happened to the various feminist and queer attempts of adopting, of resignifying and deconstructing the concepts of perversion and hysteria? In which way are hysteria and perversion linked? What does the case study of Dora teach us about sex and gender? How can we understand perversion and hysteria from a queer perspective? And finally, how can we think a productive relation between Psychoanalysis and Queer Theory? Two 'disciplines' that share a common interest – both are dealing with questions concerning subjectivity, identity, sexuality and gender – but that are also fundamentally different from each other: the first is a clinical discipline, the second the critical product of political activism.

* * *

In feminist and postmodern theories hysteria and perversion are interpreted as subversive forces, which undermine the hegemonic, heteronormative and patriarchal order, while at the same time being analyzed as discursive practices that inscribe power into bodies and subjects. In addition, hysteria and perversion compete with each other concerning the 'radicalism' of their subversive force.

Hysteria particularly has a long tradition of being misused for women's suppression. Long before Breuer and Freud's *Studies on Hysteria* was published, many medical and psychological publications were addressing this issue, concluding that intellectual exercise causes hysteria and recommended that women should be kept away from such damaging influences. By the end of the 19th century scientific publications on femininity as well as diagnoses of hysteria reached their peak. Women's bodies and minds were regarded as infused with nature and sexual drives and thus, were perceived as requiring particular attention and control. Women were considered to be sexualized through and

---

[4] Ibid., p. 119.
[5] S. Freud, 'Fragment of an Analysis of a Case of Hysteria' (1905 [1901]), *SE* 7, p. 13.

through, while the actual existence of their sexual organs was negated and imagined only as a small penis. Woman was not perceived as sexual subject but, rather, as *sexuality* itself.[6] Since the 1970s feminist thinkers, primarily difference feminists and feminist deconstructivists, started to re-appropriate hysteria in order to regain woman as subject and to argue for a female sexuality beyond patriarchal definitions.

In *This Sex Which Is Not One* the feminist philosopher and psychoanalyst Luce Irigaray interprets hysteria as that which "*speaks* in the mode of a paralyzed gestural faculty, of an impossible and also a forbidden speech (…)"[7] For Irigaray, hysteria mimes, reproduces, and thereby deformes the masculine discourse on femininity: "To play with mimesis is thus, for a woman, to try to recover the place of her exploitation by discourse, without allowing herself to be simply reduced to it."[8] Irigaray's reading of hysteria as mimesis restores women as subjects of discourse – contrary to patriarchy which turns them into an object. In *Sorties*, Hélène Cixous addresses Dora to inscribe her as subject: "It is you Dora, you, who cannot be tamed, the poetic body, the true 'mistress' of the Signifier."[9] Similar to Irigaray, for Cixous women cannot exist as subjects within the patriarchal symbolic order. There is no representation of women, because that which is represented is always already mediated by the phallus. The 'female' as independent entity beyond the phallogocentric law has been erased; woman only exists as the negative of man, as lack, as passivity, as silence. Thus the other 'female', the 'woman' which exists outside of phallogocentrism cannot be defined – not only does she not yet exist, there also is no 'nature' or 'essence' of woman. Woman, according to Irigaray and Cixous, has to be discovered, developed, inscribed into language in order to be able to signify within the symbolic.[10] This is the woman to

---

[6] Ch. von Braun, *Nicht Ich, Logik – Lüge – Libido*. Frankfurt/M.: Verlag Neue Kritik, 1999, p. 68.
[7] L. Irigaray, 'Questions', *This Sex Which is Not One*. New York: Cornell University Press, 1985, p. 136.
[8] L. Irigaray, 'The Power of Discourse', *This Sex Which is Not One*, p. 76.
[9] H. Cixous, 'Sorties', in: H. Cixous & C. Clément (Eds.), *The Newly Born Women*, Minneapolis: University of Minnesota Press, 2008, p. 95.
[10] The question has been raised among feminists whether hysteria is already an act of feminist resistance and thus symbolic or a kind of pre-feminism that has not yet been put into words and thus remains within the imaginary. Some aspects of this debate can be found in Hélène Cixous' and Catherine Clément's conversation in *The Untenable* where Clément states: "Listen, you love Dora, but to me she never seemed a revolutionary character," and Cixous answers: "I don't give a damn about Dora; I don't fetishize her. She is the name of a certain force, which makes the little circus not work anymore." H. Cixous & C. Clément, 'The Untenable', in: *The Newly Born Women*, p. 157.

come.¹¹ Juliet Mitchell interprets hysteria and femininity in a similar fashion:

> "Femininity is, therefore, in part a repressed condition that can only be secondarily acquired in a distorted form. It is because it is repressed that femininity is so hard to comprehend both within and without psychoanalytic investigation – it returns in symptoms, such as hysteria. In the body of the hysteric, male and female, lies the feminine protest against the law of the father. But what is repressed is both the representation of the desire and the prohibition against it: there is nothing 'pure' or 'original' about it."¹²

According to Christina von Braun, cultural practices as well as traditional theories on hysteria try to annihilate the sexual female body, while the hysterics make themselves an embodiment of the destroyed sexual being in order to gain her body back.¹³ Dora's adoption of her mother's symptoms – absence of voice, difficulties of breathing and a catarrh in her abdomen – creates in von Braun's interpretation a language between mother and daughter and marks the refusal of the mother tongue to be absorbed by the father tongue.¹⁴

The question of loss plays an important part in all these feminist debates on hysteria. But contrary to the traditional psychoanalytic perspective it is not about the loss of the penis/phallus. Different from the mainstream feminist debates on hysteria but nevertheless centering on the question of loss, Teresa de Lauretis, in *The Practice of Love: Lesbian Sexuality and Perverse Desire*, develops a conception of female homosexuality and female desire as independent from masculinity. She understands female homosexuality as linked to a perverse, fetishistic desire that fantasmatically tries to recover the lost female body. For de Lauretis the woman is not castrated because she lacks the penis/phallus but because she has lost the female body image: "The fantasmatic object in lesbian object-choice is not the mother, I maintain, but the subject's own body-image, the denied and wished-for female body which castration threatens with

---

[11] See, H. Cixous, 'The Laugh of the Medusa', *Signs*, Vol. 1, No.4, 1976, p. 875-893 and L. Irigaray, 'When Our Lips Speak Together', *This Sex Which Is Not One*, L. Irigaray (Ed.). New York: Cornell University Press, 1985, p. 205-218.
[12] J. Mitchell, *Psychoanalysis and Feminism*. New York: Basic Books, 2000, p. 404.
[13] Von Braun, *Nicht Ich, Logik – Lüge – Libido*, p. 57.
[14] Ibid., p. 195.

non-existence (…)".[15] In 'Fragment of an Analysis of a Case of Hysteria', Dora speaks of the 'adorable white body' of Frau K.[16] Dora may desire Frau K., she may as well identify with her, but in addition an image of the female body might emerge that could mirror a 'female' subject, establish a female imaginary and thus bring 'woman' into existence. Contrary to Freud, de Lauretis argues that the fetish is not a sign of deficient development but is constructed retroactively, often using signs of masculinity, not because of the so called masculinity-complex, but because masculinity explicitly "signif[ies] sexual desire toward women" and "much more consequential" the "wish for a female body-ego".[17] Perverse desire for de Lauretis is not a subversive force but rather bound to the disavowal of the lack (the narcissistic loss of a body-image).

In contrast to de Lauretis, Georges Bataille's approach to perversion contains a transgressive moment. He does not analyze hidden or unconscious anxieties, wishes and traumas in order to integrate them, instead, he transforms them into conscious perverse and obscene images. Bataille, as Schaffner puts it, "celebrates perversion as a means of deep communication, as a path to the experience of community and the continuity of being. Perversion is not the symptom but the cure (…)".[18] Following this interpretation, perversion seems to grant access to a particular truth of being. Feminist historian and film theorist Kaja Silverman interprets perversion as that which goes beyond sexual difference and which "strips sexuality of all functionality, whether biological or social; in an even more extreme fashion than 'normal' sexuality, it puts the body and the world of objects to uses that have nothing whatever to do with any kind of 'immanent' design or purpose."[19] Furthermore, in Silverman's interpretation perversion subverts binary oppositions which are foundational for our culture, for example food/excrement, pleasure/pain, human/animal, life/death, … Nevertheless, Silverman argues that perversions are not subversive *per se*. For the philosopher Jonathan Dollimore perversion is a "transgressive agency inseparable from a dynamic intrinsic to social process."[20] Similarly to Silverman, he interprets perversion as

---

[15] T. de Lauretis, *The Practice of Love. Lesbian Sexuality and Perverse Desire.* Bloomington: Indiana University Press, 1994, p. 288. See also, T. Dean and Ch. Lane, 'Homosexuality and Psychoanalysis: An Introduction', in: *Homosexuality and Psychoanalysis*, T. Dean & Ch. Lane (Eds.), Chicago: University of Chicago Press, 2001, p. 23.
[16] Freud, 'Fragment', p. 61.
[17] De Lauretis, *The Practice of Love*, p. 264.
[18] A. K. Schaffner, *Modernism and Perversion: Sexual Deviance in Sexology and Literature, 1850-1930*. Basingstoke: Palgrave, 2012, p. 251.
[19] K. Silverman, *Male Subjectivity at the Margins*. New York: Psychology Press, 1992, p. 187.
[20] J. Dollimore, *Sexual Dissidence: Augustine to Wilde, Freud to Foucault*. Oxford: Oxford University Press, 1991, p. 33.

a refusal of hegemonic principles of culture, such as sexual difference, the law of the father or heterosexuality.[21] Adopting Michel Foucault's understanding of power, perversion for Dollimore is produced – but at the same time it is inscribed at the heart of the oedipal situation and it might therefore carry transgressive and subversive forces within it.[22] Teresa de Lauretis criticizes this perspective on perversion as 'romanticizing', especially what Dollimore calls the "insurrectionary nature of the perversions."[23]

Paul B. Preciado's concept of 'contra-sexuality' tries to establish a productive rather than a repressive form of sexuality that goes hand in hand with the deconstruction of the sexed and gendered body. He understands sexuality as technology and its elements (bodies, sexes, identities, …) as machines, products, tools, gadgets, devices, prostheses, programs, energies, mechanisms, interruptions, connections and much more.[24] The dildo marks a central figure within his theoretical approach: it is the invention of the dildo that determines, according to Preciado, the penis as cause of sexual difference. It represents an original reality, which retroactively creates the penis as origin. From the perspective of deconstruction the dildo precedes the penis.

> "Gender is like the dildo, because they are both more than imitation. Its carnal plasticity destabilizes the distinction between the imitated and the imitator, between truth and representation of the truth, between reference and the referent, between nature and the artificial, between the sexual organs and the practices of sex. Gender could result from a sophisticated technology that manufactures sexual bodies."[25]

Preciado views sexuality, gender, bodies, … as prosthetic forms of technology. Thus, from a psychoanalytic point of view, he proposes an understanding of sexuality that could be called perverse – for Preciado there is only perversion and nothing beyond. This perspective is very close to Freud's deconstruction of perversion as pathology (to be discussed later in this essay) – a perspective that is much more radical, I would suggest, than perceiving perversion as a kind of repressed sexuality that simply needs to/must be freed. Differences notwithstanding, most feminist and gender theories on hysteria and perversion

---

[21] Ibid., p. 198.
[22] See, J. Campbell, *Arguing with the Pallus. Feminist, Queer and Postcolonial Theory. A Psychoanalytic Contribution*. London: Zed Books, 2000, p. 140.
[23] De Lauretis, *The Practice of Love*, p. 26.
[24] B. Preciado, *Kontrasexuelles Manifest*. Berlin: b_books, 2003, p. 11.
[25] http://autonomies.org/ar/2012/11/the-rebellion-of-bodies-beatriz-preciado/ (accessed on 21-3-2017).

argue for a transformation of the established sexual arrangement – they try to destabilize the dominance of the phallus and the hegemonic order of sexual difference.

In the following I will critically discuss the interpretation of perversion as subversive force based in repression and – in a final step – suggest that the subversive potential attributed to hysteria is more far-reaching. Although Queer Theory has a high affinity for perversions, it is my aim to theoretically link feminist discourses on hysteria with queer perspectives and suggest that it is hysteria (and not perversion), which can be brought in a productive relationship with queer perspectives even if it is both a product of discourse and a force that transgresses it.

* * *

Michael Foucault, in *The History of Sexuality*, also addressed the issue of hysteria and perversion, viewing both as actively produced by culture and discourse. Against the common belief that perversions are repressed and have to be freed in order to create a progressive, non-restrictive, liberated society, Foucault understands perversion as a product and a medium of power. According to his approach, it is perversion which enables power to effectively operate in the field of the psycho-sexual. Thus, perversion is not repressed at all, rather perversions are 'implanted' into the subjects.[26]

Freud's view of perversion changed over time, which resulted in different concepts of perversion. In his case study on Dora ('Fragment') Freud writes:

"All psychoneurotics are persons with strongly marked perverse tendencies, which have been repressed in the course of their development and have become unconscious. (…) Psychoneuroses are, so to speak, the negative of perversions. (…) The motive forces leading to the formation of hysterical symptoms draw their strength not only from repressed normal sexuality but also from unconscious perverse activities."[27]

Both in the *Three Essays on the Theory of Sexuality* and in the 'Fragment' Freud links perversion and hysteria – the latter seems to be the result of the repression of the first. This may have contributed to later readings of perversion as a kind of 'positive' sexuality that should not be repressed but freed. This simplification of the Freudian concept of perversion – linked to neurosis as its negative form

---

[26] Foucault, *The History of Sexuality. Volume I*, p. 36.
[27] Freud, 'Fragment', pp. 50-51.

– led to the assumption that perversion could be interpreted as subversive political strategy. In this reading perversion exceeds all norms and laws without any conflicts that lead to repression and it remains outside the effects of power. In his later works, for example in his discussion of fetishism in 'An Outline of Psycho-Analysis', Freud explains that perversions are not simply the 'positive' side of neurosis but are distinguished from neurosis by a specific and complex structure of defenses, such as disavowal of reality, splitting of the ego, etc.[28] In addition to this rather structural explanation of perversion Freud, in the case study on Dora, describes perverse acts, such as the sexual use of lips. In that these so called 'perverse acts' are part of every human sexuality Freud moved on to a deconstruction of sexual perversion as pathology. Later commentators confirm this view. Following Steven Marcus' introduction to the *Three Essays* in 1975 Teresa de Lauretis subsumes that Freud's "theory of sexuality is based on both representations and practices of sex that are, to a greater or lesser degree, 'perverse'".[29] Jean Laplanche and Jean-Bertrand Pontalis emphasize that the "(s)o-called normal sexuality cannot be seen as an *a priori* aspect of human nature" and that "Freud's originality lies in the fact that he used the existence of perversion as a weapon with which to throw the traditional definition of sexuality into question."[30] Freud can be read as progressive thinker in this respect: he deconstructs the notion of perversion as pathology and paves the way for later queer re-readings.[31]

* * *

---

[28] S. Freud, 'An Outline of Psycho-Analysis' (1940 [1938]), *SE* 23.

[29] De Lauretis, *The Practice of Love*, p. 10.

[30] J. Laplanche & J.-B. Pontalis, *The Language of Psycho-Analysis*. New York: Norton, 1973, p. 307.

[31] In spite of the revolutionary elements within Freud's thinking, there are also conservative aspects. At one point in the 'Fragment' he explains the normality of perversions, directly followed by the claim that perversions are the reason for inhibited development: "The sexual life of each one of us extends to a slight degree—now in this direction, now in that— beyond the narrow lines imposed as the standard of normality. The perversions are neither bestial nor degenerate in the emotional sense of the word. They are a development of germs all of which are contained in the undifferentiated sexual disposition of the child, and which, by being suppressed or by being diverted to higher, asexual aims—by being 'sublimated' — are destined to provide the energy for a great number of our cultural achievements. When, therefore, any one has *become* a gross and manifest pervert, it would be more correct to say that he has *remained* one, for he exhibits a certain stage of *inhibited development*." Freud, 'Fragment, p. 50.

From a Lacanian perspective hysteria and perversion cannot be defined or diagnosed on grounds of particular symptoms, but represent a specific mode of being in relation to the symbolic order. This implies a different view regarding the subversive potential of perversions. According to Slavoj Žižek, who follows Lacan in this point, one could question perversion as subversion. For Žižek, hysteria is much more subversive than perversions. Žižek points out that an understanding of perversion as "the other side of neuroses", would lead to the erasure of the key concept of psychoanalysis – the unconscious.[32]

At first glance, following Freud's thesis of neurosis as the negative of perversions, as discussed above, it seems to be clear, that the perverts openly realize and practice what the hysterics repress. As Žižek explains, the pervert believes, that he or she knows the truth of the secret fantasies while the hysteric remains questioning the truth of secrets. This is why Žižek can claim that – while living our perverse fantasies – we 'loose' our unconscious. The "pervert precludes the unconscious" because he is sure he knows the truth of what brings *jouissance*. The hysteric is the one who doubts, who repeatedly questions her relation to the other: "Hysteria is not simply the battleground between secret desires and symbolic prohibitions; it also, and above all, articulates the gnawing doubt whether secret desires really contain what they promise – whether our inability to enjoy really hinges only on symbolic prohibitions."[33] Žižek concludes that the pervert's discourse sustains the predominant discourse, while the hysterics, on the other hand, are truly radical, because they question whether those secret fantasies are really the repressed secrets of a subject or a culture.

This argument is supported by Freud himself, who claimed, that only hysteria and psychosis – not perversion – offer a way to the unconscious[34] and it also conforms with Freud's understanding of perversions as based on specific defense mechanisms such as splitting.[35] Thus Žižek can state that the acting out in perversion is darkening the unconscious.

Those feminist discourses discussing hysteria – e. g. Hélène Cixous' approach – are not rejecting the potentiality of perversion as subversion but they are emphasizing in particular the subversive potential of the unconscious which cannot be domesticated: "Now women return from afar, from always: from 'without,' from the heath where witches are kept alive; from below, from beyond

---

[32] S. Žižek, *The Ticklish Subject*. London: Verso, 1999, p. 247.
[33] Ibid., p. 248.
[34] Ibid.
[35] This structural, Lacanian and Žižekian notion of perversion must be differentiated from Freud's notion of perversion as aspect within every sexuality. In the latter case one cannot claim in general that the unconscious is 'lost' or precluded. It could but must not be the case.

'culture'; (...) Here they are, returning, arriving over and again, because the unconscious is impregnable."[36] Psychoanalyst and queer theorist Eve Watson also perceives the unconscious as subversive moment, although it contains the signifiers of the symbolic order, but in addition it "precludes the possibility of a categorical or unproblematic identity".[37]

The hysteric was and is considered as the heroine of feminist protest that resists sexual norms, as the one who finds a way to speak where patriarchy has silenced her, as the one who saves woman's "sexuality from total repression and destruction."[38] Hysteria furthermore represents "woman in all her force", it makes her an "element that disturbs."[39] Talking about the case of Dora Hélène Cixous writes: "Dora seemed to me to be the one who resisted the system, the one who cannot stand that the family and society are founded on the body of women, on bodies despised, rejected, bodies that are humiliating once they have been used."[40]

One of the main goals of the feminist approach has been to bring the excluded, rejected, the feminine, the black, the dark, et cetera of a society or culture back into discourse and into the symbolic order. Following this agenda the discourse of the hysteric is viewed as passage to this excluded territory. This does not mean that the unconscious is annulled, rather the unconscious is perceived as vivid and infinite source of subversion, which at the same time should not be glorified or mystified as a primordial sphere. As I quoted Mitchell above, there is nothing "pure" or "original" within the repressed or excluded. The repressed, the excluded or the unconscious is no residuum that preserves an original or secret truth about sex, gender, or the female.

***

What are the consequences of feminists' adopting and resignifying hysteria? What does hysteria teach us about gender?

Jane Gallop turns to the connection Freud makes between hysteria and bisexuality: "Freud links hysteria to bisexuality; the hysteric identifies with members of both sexes, cannot choose one sexual identity. (...) If feminism

---

[36] Cixous, 'The Laugh of the Medusa', p. 877.
[37] E. Watson, 'Queering Psychoanalysis/Psychoanalysing Queer', in: *Annual Review of Critical Psychology* 7 (2009), p. 123.
[38] L. Irigaray, *Speculum of the other Women*. Ithaca, New York: Cornell University Press, 1985, p. 72.
[39] Cixous & Clément, 'The Untenable', pp. 254 ff.
[40] Ibid., p. 154.

is the calling into question of constraining sexual identities, then the hysteric may be a protofeminist" [41] – or: a queer activist, one could add from today's perspective. Going in a similar direction, following Freud, Claire Kahane describes a "fluidity of psychic identifications". She notes:

> "What Dora revealed was that sexual difference was a psychological problematic rather than a natural fact, that it existed within the individual psyche as well as between men and women in culture. Am I a man? Am I a woman? How is sexual identity assumed? How represented? These are the hysterical questions as Freud developed them out of the matrix of psychic bisexuality, as well as the central questions of psychoanalysis."[42]

In the case study on Dora it seems that identification and desire do not exclude each other. Dora identifies with the father she desires, just as she identifies with Frau K. whom she desires as well. Jan Campbell follows Diana Fuss' interpretation in *Identification Papers*, claiming "that desire and identification are not distinct but hopelessly entwined. Sexual identity consists of identifying with the person you desire and desiring the person with whom you identify."[43] This argument calls the simplifications of the Oedipus complex into question. Parveen Adams' discussion of Freud's case study on Dora points in a very similar direction. As she elaborates, the hysteric demonstrates that Freud's assumed opposition between object choice and identification collapses and that identification with both men and women is actually possible. Adams describes hysterical identification as characterized by oscillation between a masculine and a feminine position. For her this would have serious consequences for our understanding of the Oedipus complex and the development of masculinity and femininity: "For if it turns out that the identification which produces sexual difference within the Oedipus complex is hysterical identification, then the resolution of the Oedipus complex cannot explain the transformation of bisexuality into a fixed sexual position."[44]

---

[41] Gallop cited by E. Showalter, 'Hysteria, Feminism and Gender', in: *S.* Gilman, H. King, R. Porte, G. S. Rousseau & E. Showalter (Eds.), *Hysteria Beyond Freud*. Berkeley: University of California Press, 1993, p. 288.
[42] Kahane, 'Introduction. Part Two', Ch. Bernheimer & C. Kahane (Eds.), *In Dora's Case. Freud – Hysteria – Feminism*. New York: Columbia University Press, 1985, p. 22.
[43] J. Campbell, *Arguing with the Pallus. Feminist, Queer and Postcolonial Theory. A Psychoanalytic Contribution*. London: Zed Books, 2000, p. 147.
[44] P. Adams, 'Per Os(cillation)', in: J. Donald (Ed.), *Psychoanalysis and Cultural Theory: Thresholds*, New York: Macmillan, 1990, p. 70.

As hysteria addresses the question of identification and desire it can be linked to contemporary queer discourses and their attempt of deconstructing fixed identities.

Following Lacan, Anne Worthington also understands the questions raised by the hysteric as questions about sex: What is a woman? What is a man? What kind of man or woman am I? Am I a woman, a man, or trans? Am I straight, gay, bisexual or queer? Worthington asks: If psychoanalysis was the answer to hysteria during the last turn of the century, isn't Queer Theory the answer to the questions of hysteria in our times?[45] I found this thesis very interesting and would like to pursue it further in order to rethink and reformulate it in a slightly different manner. I would like to argue for a productive entanglement of psychoanalysis and Queer Theory. Psychoanalysis and Queer Theory must not mutually exclude or replace each other. Postmodern approaches have offered us the promising idea of deconstructing scientific disciplines and discourses, which are no longer perceived as closed systems. Instead, I would like to follow Gilles Deleuze's and Félix Guattari's mode of thinking in plateaus as open systems. Therefore, I suggest we think the relationship between Queer Theory and psychoanalysis as entangling plateaus in order to avoid fixations and absolute truth and to open and deconstruct scientific disciplines. As Brian Massumi puts it in his preface to *A Thousand Plateaus*: "Each 'plateau' is an orchestration of crashing bricks extracted from a variety of disciplinary edifices."[46] Contrary to a discipline, a plateau rejects homogeneity but still includes a kind of composition and consistency, it is always in the middle, instead of marking the beginning or the end.[47] Following this interpretation, this essay could also be perceived as composed of plateaus instead of terminated chapters.

* * *

In my view, the epistemological figure of the plateau also promises to offer new perspectives on the discourse on hysteria that might overcome the limitations of both, Psychoanalysis and Queer Theory: Is hysteria only a woman's disease or could it also become a man's disease, or the disease of the powerless and silenced? Are the 'hysterical questions' and topics, for example the questions about sexual identity, about the body et cetera only women's questions? Elaine Showalter notes: "We might answer that the despised hysterics of yesteryear

---

[45] Cf. A. Worthington, 'Beyond Queer?', in: A. Grose (Ed.) *Hysteria Today*. London: Karnac, 2016, p. 41.

[46] B. Massumi, 'Translator's Foreword', in: G. Deleuze & F. Guattari, *A Thousand Plateaus*. Minneapolis: University of Minnesota Press, 2005, p. x.

[47] Deleuze & Guattari, *A Thousand Plateaus*, p. 21.

have been replaced by the feminist radicals of today, by contemporary women artists and poets, and by gay activists." For Showalter, hysteria is not just the disease of women and could also be linked to questions of race and suppression.[48]

Within the feminist discourse on hysteria there is another aspect that can be read together with queer perspectives: It seems that the subversive moments in the discourse of the hysteric, which are the mimetic, the fluid et cetera – aspects that, following Luce Irigaray and Hélène Cixous, challenge the predominant expectations on femininity, masculinity, identity and sexuality – found their way into Queer Theory. Within the feminist discourses of the 70s the hysteric was the figure of the burlesque, the liar. The hysteric radically questioned – and still questions – the status of the woman as object, she reclaims herself as the subject of 'femininity' and, so to speak, of 'her illness'. The hysteric is thus an artificial character. She performs, as Christina von Braun puts it, fantasies of femininity. A similar figure can be found today in queer drag-performances. As Judith Butler explains:

> "To claim that all gender is like drag, or is drag, is to suggest that 'imitation' is at the heart of the *heterosexual* project and its gender binarisms, that drag is not a secondary imitation that presupposes a prior and original gender, but that hegemonic heterosexuality is itself a constant and repeated effort to imitate its own idealizations."[49]

As Butler explains, drag performances imitate gender and illustrate the "imitative structure of gender itself".[50] Drag as gender parody demonstrates furthermore that there is no original: "the parody is *of* the very notion of an original."[51] In addition, for Butler, gender is a performance, which is falsely naturalized. Similar to von Braun's hysterics who perform "fantasies of femininity", Butler understands gender identification as constituted by a fantasy. Both the hysterics and the drag kings and queens criticize naturalized or essentialist gender identities.

For Luce Irigaray and Hélène Cixous – and this is part of the hysteric's discourse – woman is the one to come, the one not yet existing within the order of patriarchy, the one to be never fixed, always remaining fluid in her identity. Queer Theory also criticizes identities and identity politics, it argues for a transgression of identities, or thinking identities without an essence. Similar to Irigaray's and Cixous' notion of the woman to come, David Halperin writes about queer:

---

[48] Showalter, 'Hysteria, Feminism and Gender', p. 288 and 334.
[49] J. Butler, *Bodies that Matter*. Routledge, New York 1993, p. 125.
[50] J. Butler, *Gender Trouble*. Routledge, New York, 1999, p. 175.
[51] Ibid.

> "Queer is by definition *whatever* is at odds with the normal, the legitimate, the dominant. *There is nothing in particular to which it necessarily refers.* It is an identity without an essence. 'Queer' then, demarcates not a positivity but a positionality vis-à-vis the normative … (Queer) describes a horizon of possibility whose precise extent and heterogeneous scope cannot in principle be delimited in advance."[52]

Queer Theory as well as a queering perspective within psychoanalysis do not aim to resolve the 'great riddle of the sex', they keep the questions on sexuality, desire and identity on an open plateau, just as hysterics do.

---

[52] D. M. Halperin, *Saint Foucault: Toward a Gay Hagiography*. Oxford: Oxford University Press, 1995, p. 62.

Notes on the Contributors

Rachel B. Blass is a member and training analyst at the Israel Psychoanalytic Society, a member of the British Psychoanalytical Society, and professor of psychoanalysis at Heythrop College, the University of London. She is also a board member and editor of the "Controversies" section of the *International Journal of Psychoanalysis*. She has published a book and over 80 articles which deal mainly with the close study and elucidation of Freud's texts and Kleinian thinking and practice. She has lectured, taught and offered clinical seminars in many countries and her writings have been translated into fifteen languages.

Daniela Finzi is a literary and cultural scholar. She is member of the board of the Sigmund Freud Foundation and, as head of the research department of the Sigmund Freud Museum, she is in charge of the academic exhibitions, research projects and conference programme of Berggasse 19. She is also a board member of "aka – Arbeitskreis Kulturanalyse" and co-editor of the book series aka|texte and Sigmund Freuds Werke: Wiener Interdisziplinäre Kommentare. She has written on cultural theory, gender studies and Balkan studies.

Esther Hutfless is a philosopher and psychoanalyst in Vienna. She teaches at the Department of Philosophy at the University of Vienna. Her main research areas include: deconstruction, psychoanalysis, feminist philosophy, écriture féminine, and queer theory. Her publications include: *Queering Psychoanalysis. Psychoanalyse und Queer Theory * Transdisziplinäre Verschränkungen* (ed. with Barbara Zach, 2017), *Hélène Cixous. Gespräch mit dem Esel. Blind Schreiben.* (ed. with Elisabeth Schäfer, 2017).

Ulrike Kadi is a philosopher, psychiatrist and practicing psychoanalyst. She is associate professor at the Department of Psychoanalysis and Psychotherapy at the Medical University of Vienna. Her main fields are poststructuralism, psychopathology and psychoanalysis (Lacan). Most recently she has co-edited (with Sabine Schlüter and Elisabeth Skale) *Fremd. Im eigenen Haus. Sigmund-Freud-Vorlesungen 2016* (Mandelbaum 2017). She is currently leading the FWF project "Topographies of the Body. Phenomenological, Genealogical and Psychoanalytic Investigations". For further information see kadicorps.philo.at.

Ilka Quindeau is full professor of clinical psychology and psychoanalysis at Frankfurt University of Applied Sciences and associate professor at Johann Wolfgang Goethe-University Frankfurt. She is president of the Sigmund Freud Foundation in Frankfurt and also runs her own practice. Trained as a clinical psychologist and sociologist, she is now working as a training and supervising analyst in the German and International Psychoanalytical Society (DPV/IPA). She has published over 100 chapters and articles and has authored or edited several books. In 2018 she will head the International Psychoanalytic University in Berlin.

Beatriz Santos is an associate professor at the Department of Psychoanalytical Studies at Université Paris Diderot. She is a practicing psychoanalyst and a member of the International Society for Psychoanalysis and Philosophy. She writes about the possibilities of dialogues between psychoanalysis in gender studies and has recently published (with Laurie Laufer) 'Language and Vulnerability—A Lacanian Analysis of Respect' in *Frontiers in Psychology* (2017), 8:2279.

Philippe Van Haute is full professor of philosophical anthropology at Radboud University Nijmegen, and extraordinary professor at the University of Pretoria. He is a practicing psychoanalyst and was president of the Belgian School for Psychoanalysis from 2006 to 2009. He has published numerous articles and books on Freudian psychoanalysis, amongst others (with Tomas Geyskens) *A Non-Oedipal Psychoanalysis? A Clinical Anthropology of Hysteria in the Works of Freud and Lacan* (2012). Most recently he has published (with Herman Westerink) several text editions of the first edition of Freud's *Three Essays on the Theory of Sexuality*.

Herman Westerink is senior researcher and lecturer for the philosophy of religion and intercultural philosophy at the Radboud University Nijmegen and extraordinary professor at the KU Leuven. He is the vice-chair of the Advisory Board of the Sigmund Freud Foundation. He has written many books and articles on psychoanalysis, sexuality, melancholia and religion, most recently (with Philippe Van Haute) commentaries on and text editions of the first edition of Freud's *Three Essays on the Theory of Sexuality*.

Jeanne Wolff-Bernstein is a psychoanalyst in Vienna. She was president and training analyst at the Psychoanalytic Institute of Northern California (PINC), San Francisco. She teaches at the Sigmund Freud University in Vienna, at PINC and at The New York University Postdoctoral Program of Psychoanalysis and Psychotherapy. She is a member of the Wiener Arbeitskreis für Psychoanalyse. She is the chair of the Advisory Board of the Sigmund Freud Foundation in Vienna. She has written extensively on psychoanalysis and the visual arts and on the work of Jacques Lacan.

www.ingramcontent.com/pod-product-compliance
Ingram Content Group UK Ltd.
Pitfield, Milton Keynes, MK11 3LW, UK
UKHW021834140426
5217IPUK00021B/1448